HEART BYPASS:

WHAT EVERY PATIENT <u>MUST</u> KNOW

HEART BYPASS:

WHAT EVERY PATIENT <u>MUST</u> KNOW

by Gloria Hochman

Foreword by
Dr. William Likoff

Introduction by
Dr. Denton A. Cooley

ST. MARTIN'S PRESS   NEW YORK

For information, write: St. Martin's Press,
175 Fifth Avenue, New York, N.Y. 10010
Manufactured in the United States of America

Library of Congress Cataloging in Publication Data

Hochman, Gloria.
   Heart bypass, what every patient must know.

   1. Aortocoronary bypass. 2. Surgery—Popular
works. I. Title.
RD598.H58   617'.412   81–21481
ISBN 0–312–36597–7   AACR2

Design by Kingsley Parker

10 9 8 7 6 5 4 3 2

The publisher would like to thank The National Heart,
Lung, and Blood Institute for its cooperation, and for
the use of the illustrations on pages 34 and 40.

For my extraordinary family,
    especially

for Stan with love
for Charlotte with devotion
for Anndee whose smile lights up my life

This book was written in memory of my uncle

Bernard S. Ochman

who made me believe, a long time ago, that
a woman could be anything she wanted to be.

CONTENTS

FOREWORD

In simpler times a physician was not expected to reveal matters of substance to a patient. Since knowledge of most illnesses was neither profound nor accurate and scarcely worth transmitting, the ethics of this lack of meaningful communication were seldom debated. Indeed, the barrier of silence separating physician and patient was viewed as a hallmark of professionalism, not an abridgement of individual rights.

Over the years this convention has changed remarkably. As knowledge of health problems increased, so did the need to share that information with the laity. Not the least of the reasons was the common experience that the informed patient is the more understanding, the more cooperative and the more able to contribute to recovery. This also holds for members of families who become involved because of the presence in their midst of someone who is ill. Today a policy of open discussion has almost entirely erased the secrecy of the past.

The transmission of knowledge regarding health sciences to the laity is an art form of itself. To be meaningful, information must be factual and comprehensive. Above all, it must be stated clearly, accurately, and understandably. Obviously, all of this is not readily achieved because knowledge in the health sciences is usually incomplete and beclouded by uncertain theory and bias which cannot be translated appropriately for the uninformed and untrained.

Gloria Hochman has mastered the difficulties of the task. Unquestionably what contributes to the timeliness and importance of her book is the endemic nature and incidence of coronary heart disease in western civilization and the smoldering controversy regarding the place of surgery in treatment.

Coronary heart disease evolves as a result of the deposition of cellular debris along the interior lining of arteries which nourish the heart muscle. The process is known as atherosclerosis. While the specific cause of atherosclerosis is unknown, there are a number of so-called risk factors which are believed to increase its likelihood or acceleration. Included among them are significant hypertension, diabetes, abnormally high concentrations of circulating fats or lipids, cigarette smoking, lack of appropriate exercise, and more remotely, obesity.

Perhaps the most important risk factor is genetically endowed and involves a multi-factorial error in blood clotting as well as fat metabolism. It is imperative in evaluating risk factors not to confuse theory with fact. Decisions to alter fundamental life-styles in the interest of minimizing the progress of atherosclerosis must be made with that clearly in mind.

Atherosclerosis progressively narrows the internal caliber of the coronary arteries. The speed with which this takes place varies greatly from individual to individual. When the internal caliber of one or many arteries is reduced by at least 50 percent, nourishment of the heart muscle supplied by such arteries is materially diminished and symptoms may appear. The nature of the complaints may differ greatly and include shortness of breath, unwarranted fatigue, sensation of rapid heart beating, and chest discomfort classically known as angina pectoris.

Although more than two centuries have passed since the first clinical description of angina was published, time and experience have not materially challenged the accuracy of the first account which underscored the relation of discomfort to physical and emotional stress and its abatement with rest. Indeed, even the risk of sudden death during an attack was clearly pointed out as well as, by contrast, the fact that it was possible for the afflicted to enjoy many years of productive life. Modern statistics support the latter view. It is estimated that as many as 40 percent of individuals with angina may live fifteen years or more.

A number of adjectives are used to better define the variations in the clinical pattern of angina pectoris which are commonly encountered. The term "stable angina" suggests the syndrome is predictable rather than progressively worse in frequency or severity. Recent onset of angina is identified as "angina de nova" while a relentless progression in severity is called "crescendo" and "intractable" or "unstable."

Although the prospects are increasingly good for most patients, a severe compromise in the internal caliber of one or more coronary arteries results in a critical decrease in blood flow to a section of the heart muscle leading to its death. The patient does not necessarily die. Indeed, in the majority of instances the individual recovers but the segment of heart muscle thereafter either fails to contract or does so in an abnormal or impaired fashion. The technical term "myocardial infarction" is used to describe the event. The laity generally speaks of the episode as a "heart attack."

Although a heart attack may occur suddenly without symptomatic warning, it must be emphasized that it is the result of a slowly developing disease process, coronary artery atherosclerosis. There is reasonable evidence that several processes may precipitate complete closure of a narrowed vessel.

First among them is spasm or a sudden constriction of the involved artery. The cause of this exaggerated functional narrowing is not understood, but its effect may be devastating. Secondly, sluggish blood flow through the narrowed artery may result in the formation of a clot which is superimposed upon the arterial debris and totally occludes the vessel.

Modern advances in diagnostic techniques assist materially in defining the extent of the arterial disease. The gold standard for such an inquiry is the coronary arteriogram which depicts the internal caliber of the vessels nourishing the cardiac muscle. In addition, the distribution of blood flow to the heart and the contractile characteristics of the muscle can be analyzed by scanning techniques using radioactive material. The function of the electrical system of the heart is defined by the ordinary electrocardiogram.

Modern treatment programs reduce disability from angina and also decrease the risk of death following a "heart attack." Drugs currently in common use include agents that decrease the work of the heart, dilate the coronary arteries, as well as prevent the influx of calcium into the arterial cell which, at least theoretically, decreased the likelihood of spasm.

Heart Bypass: What Every Patient Must *Know* is an exciting perspective of the surgical treatment of coronary heart disease. The technique commonly employed involves the insertion of a vein graft (taken from the patient's leg) above and below the narrowed coronary artery thus bypassing the vascular obstruction. There is considerable evidence to suggest that 85 percent of those suffering from angina are relieved of their disability by the operation. However, there is some question whether life itself is extended.

The decision as to whether surgery should be employed is based upon a number of considerations including the severity and location of the arterial blockages, the resultant disability, the natural history of that particular structural and functional problem and the comparative risks and benefits one can expect from medical and surgical treatment. In the vast majority of instances, surgery is favored only after a reasonable medical program has failed. However, an occasional physician favors surgery as the initial therapeutic mode particularly in an effort to prevent a heart attack when the narrowed artery threatens blood flow to a large section of the myocardium.

The pursuit of understanding is a noble task. At times it is a precarious enterprise. However, in the field of health sciences it is particularly rewarding. *Heart Bypass* is a fine opportunity to achieve a worthwhile goal.

—Dr. William Likoff
President and Chief
Executive Officer,
Hahnemann Medical
College and Hospital

≡ ACKNOWLEDGMENTS

It would not have been possible for me to write a book of this complexity without the cooperation, encouragement and support of countless physicians and surgeons and their secretaries; patients; my professional colleagues; my friends; and family.

Heart Bypass grew out of an article that I wrote for the Sunday Magazine *Today* (published by the *Philadelphia Inquirer*), an article that came to be because a friend, Bob Epp, convinced me that it was needed. Response from readers was evidence of how much it was needed.

It is my hope that those of you who read this book will understand more fully and be better able to make thoughtful decisions about heart bypass surgery, the fastest-growing operation in medical history.

My sincere thanks and gratitude to the following people for sharing their time, experience and expertise with me so that heart patients, their friends and families might pursue their health care more perceptively.

Special thanks to Dr. Gerald Lemole, who was patient with me when I didn't know an angiogram from an angioplasty; to Dr. Floyd Loop, who has held my hand every step of the way; to Dr. Horace MacVaugh, who guided me through a coronary bypass operation; to Dr. Denton Cooley for working with me throughout the preparation of this book and for taking the time to write a splendid introduction to *Heart Bypass;* to Dr. William Likoff, who has written an inspiring foreword for my book; to Dr. Vladir

Maranhao, whose heart is as big as his hands are skilled; to Dr. Robert Katz for taking my midnight telephone calls; to Drs. Willis Hurst and Richard Helfant for all of the hours they gave me; to Dr. Harold Rutenberg for being a wonderful doctor and a compassionate human being; to Dr. Isadore Rosenfeld for his insight and guidance; and to Dr. Leonard Davitch for his counsel, his judgment and his friendship.

To my editor, Bob Miller, who urged me to write *Heart Bypass,* who has given me the benefit of his skill and support and who has always been there when I needed him.

To Ruth Sherman for typing my manuscript and to Joan Spivack for her special help with research.

To David Boldt, in whose magazine this project began, and who makes writing, for me, a privilege and a pleasure; and to Scott DeGarmo who helped me understand why I had to become a writer.

To my parents, Sarah and Al Honickman, and my mother-in-law, Rose Hochman, who think that everything I write is spectacular, even if it's a note to the milkman; to my grandparents, Ethel and Samuel Ochman, who gave me love and strength; to Fred, Bryan, and Scott; to Milton, Kenny, and Marc; and to Stuart, whose determination and achievements make me very proud.

To Dr. Sariel Ablaza, Peggy Anderson, Dr. Joseph P. Atkins, Jr., Dr. John Blady, Patricia Bradley, Ruth Borock, Dr. Herbert Benson, Dr. Lamberto G. Bentivoglio, Claire Berman, Dr. Martial G. Bourassa, Dr. Eugene Braunwald, Dr. A.C. Breuer, Dr. Gerald Berenson, Dr. Bruce Gregory Brown, Dr. W. Virgil Brown, Dr. Henry Buchwald, Dr. Harold Buttram, Dr. Lucien Campeau, Dr. William Castelli, Dr. Bernard Chaitman, Dr. Thomas Chalmers, Dr. Norman Clarke, Jr., Jessie Clements, Dr. Jay Cohen, Dr. C. Richard Conti, Dr. George Crile, Dr. Timothy A.

DeRouen, Dr. Michael Ellis DeBakey, Dr. Katherine Detre, Terry Dezzl, Dr. George Diamond, Dr. Charles T. Dotter, Paula Dranov, Milton Eisenberg, Bob Epp, Dr. Stephen E. Epstein, Dr. Rene G. Favaloro, Dr. James Forrester, Dr. Meyer Friedman, Dr. Peter Frommer, Dr. Robert L. Frye, Dr. Robert E. Gerhardt, Dr. H. Edward Garrett, Barbara Gleeson, Debbie Goldberg, Judith Goldstein, Dr. Garry F. Gordon, Dr. Claude Grondin, Ronald Gross, Tania Grossinger, Martha Grossman, Dr. Harvey W. Gruchow, Dr. Lloyd Grumbles, Dr. Andreas Grüntzig, Dr. Phillip Harris, Dr. K.E. Hammermeister, Aileen Hochman, Dr. William L. Holmes, Dr. Thomas James, Carolyn Johnson and her staff, Dr. W. Dudley Johnson, Dr. Melvin P. Judkins, Dr. William B. Kannel, Mimsye Katz, Dr. Kenneth Kent, Alice Kiel, Carol Kleiman, Dr. N.T. Kouchoukos, Kathie Kotsay, Dr. Peter Kuo, Chris Land, Dr. Gerald M. Lawrie, Dr. Robert Levy, Howard Lewis, Library staff at Philadelphia College of Physicians, Patrick M. McGrady, Jr., Dr. Henry D. McIntosh, Dr. Robert W. Mahley, Dr. Jack C. Manley, Dr. Thomas Meaney, Dr. Donald Miller, Jr., Maureen Mino, Dr. Michael Mock, Dr. Arno Motulsky, Tim Mulligan, Dr. Marvin Murphy, Dr. David T. Nash, Loretta Schwartz-Nobel, Dr. Albert Oberman, York Onnen, Dr. Earl S. Perrigo, Dr. Philip Podrid, Nathan Pritikin, Mae Richard, Dr. Alfred Rimm, Dr. William C. Roberts, Dr. Robert Rosati, Dr. Ray Rosenman, Dr. George G. Rowe, Stephen Rubin, Dr. Thomas F. Santilli, Kitty Sass, Dr. Henry S. Sawin, Dodi Schultz, Dr. Richard Shekelle, Dr. John Speer Schroeder, Dr. A. Mitchell Smith, Dr. Bernard Sobel, Dr. F. Mason Sones, Jr., Gerald Spivack, Dr. Simon Stertzer, Carroll Stoner, Dr. Timothy Takaro, Leonard Tose, Joseph Taylor, Dr. Edward Viner, Dr. Paul Walinsky, Graham W. Ward, Dr. Redford B. Williams, Jr., Dr. Roger R. Williams, Dr. Donald C. Wukasch, Dolores Ziff.

And to Bernard and Fred P., Vincent D., Frank M.,
Loring C.; to the men and women of the Zipper Club of
Philadelphia; and to all of the other patients and their
families who shared their most private experiences and
feelings with me in the hope that they could offer support,
inspiration and comfort to others.

PREFACE

Fred and Bernard P. are brothers. Fred is fifty-four; Bernard, fifty-eight. Their father, Joseph, died of a heart attack when he was Bernard's age. Both Fred and Bernard have coronary artery disease, which has been painful, frightening and, at times, incapacitating.

Three years ago, Bernard underwent open-heart surgery. He chose to have the operation because "the quality of my life was important to me. I didn't want to spend the rest of my days not being able to be active and doing all of the things I like to do."

Fred says, "There's no way they're going to get me on that table and saw me down the middle like a chicken. Nothing I've heard or read has convinced me that surgery will do any good anyway. I'll take my chances."

The brothers are two of an estimated 4 million people in this country who have coronary artery disease. Many of them suffer from symptoms commonly known as *angina pectoris,* a strangling pain in the chest. Each year, more than 100,000 of these men and women have sought relief on the operating table. Others cannot or will not have the surgery. Their conditions are managed through a regimen of medication and, sometimes, through dramatic changes in the way they live.

Often the decision about whether or not to have the surgery is up to the patients. It is they who must decide, with their doctors and their families, the route they wish to follow. It is they who must ultimately weigh the benefits against the risks. And it is they who must understand the answers to such questions as:

- Why do I have coronary artery disease?
- Why are so many people with the condition opting for an operation?
- Why is the operation so controversial?
- Will it cure my disease? Will it prolong my life?
- How important is the "right" doctor?
- What is a heart catheterization? How do I know if I need one?
- What is the operation like? What are the risks?
- What will my life be like after the surgery?
- Are there alternatives to an operation that might work for me?

We hope that the information in this book, which was prepared with the cooperation of many of the country's leading physicians, cardiologists and cardiac surgeons, will help patients and their families make better-informed and more thoughtful decisions about one of the most critical dilemmas they may ever face.

≡ INTRODUCTION

These passions, simple but overwhelmingly
strong, have governed my life: the search
for knowledge and an unbearable pity for
the suffering of mankind.

—BERTRAND RUSSELL
1872–1970

Current statistics reveal heart disease causes more deaths
than any other disorder or disease and probably more
than all others combined. Then why doesn't the average
person—even a so-called "educated" one—know more
about the subject? For one reason, most individuals com-
placently consider that knowledge of disease is the responsibility of the physician, and when advice is needed,
the doctor should provide it on request. For another, a
suitable or reliable source of information may not be readily available. This book, compiled through research and
extensive interviews by Gloria Hochman, is an effort to
satisfy the second need.

Angina pectoris has affected human beings for centuries, but only in the past few decades has the condition
been clearly understood. The myocardium, or heart muscle—like other muscles in the body—is dependent upon
the nutritional support provided by small arteries for its
viability and normal function. Is it not curious that an
organ through which liters of blood pass every minute
derives no support from that huge volume? The heart
depends entirely upon the several hundred cubic centi-
meters of blood that pass through two matchstick-sized

coronary arteries. When those arteries occlude completely, the consequences may be "heart attack" or myocardial infarction. If extensive or untreated, this condition may result in immediate death or prolonged disability. Other muscles of the body suffer similar insults as their blood supply is reduced. For example, when the arteries supplying blood to the lower extremities become narrowed, walking or running produces muscular cramps or pain known as "intermittent claudication." When inadequately supplied with blood, the intestines, after a meal, cause a painful condition similar to claudication known as abdominal angina. The logical solution to such physiological deficiency is to supply more blood to the ischemic, or blood-starved, organ.

In the past, the medical profession has sought ways to accomplish this purpose through medicinal and surgical means. The internist or cardiologist approaches this supply-and-demand problem of cardiac blood either by reducing the demand or increasing the supply. The demand may be reduced by slowing the heart rate or reducing the workload by rest or with certain drugs, such as propranolol or the recently introduced calcium inhibitors. Pharmacologically, the blood supply may be increased by using vascular dilators such as nitroglycerin or other nitrate compounds. In the past, surgeons have participated in these attempts to decrease the demand and increase the blood supply; most of these efforts were only partially effective and such techniques rightfully did not receive universal acceptance and have since been discarded.

Introduction of myocardial revascularization by direct surgical bypass, however, has changed completely and for the better the treatment of patients with angina pectoris in a positive and meaningful way. The diagnostic test which has made possible this direct approach to the problem is the selective coronary arteriogram. It provides a clear and accurate assessment of the location and extent of the obstruction, and permits the cardiologist and surgeon to select patients who could benefit from surgery and to plan a logical surgical approach based upon the precise location of the bypassable arteries. In contrast to the formerly employed techniques, this approach has accomplished a success rate supported by objective proof of the efficacy by objective studies done after operation. Most reports from major centers where several thousand bypass operations have been performed reveal that significant or complete relief of angina pectoris occurs in more than 90 percent of patients.

This book is a review of the present status of the coronary bypass operation, presenting both pro and con attitudes, and opinions of the medical profession. It provides an excellent reference source for the layman, for the patient, and even for the medical profession at large. Mrs. Hochman has written an informative and highly useful book.

—Denton A. Cooley, M.D.
Surgeon-in-Chief
Texas Heart Institute
Houston, Texas

1

WHAT IS ANGINA PECTORIS, AND WHY DO I HAVE IT?

Bernard P., a businessman who lives in Cherry Hill, New Jersey, had a heart attack fifteen years ago. For six or seven years afterward, he had no symptoms and was able to live a normal, active life. But about five years ago he began to feel a little discomfort in his chest. He describes it as a tightness and pressure in the middle of his chest, just behind the breastbone, whenever he became agitated.

It didn't happen often, maybe three or four times a year. Then it began to occur more frequently, whenever he did anything even slightly exerting. Bernard is in the shoe business, and even when he lifted a couple of shoe boxes, he would get the pain. If he walked up the steps too quickly, the pain would come. Sometimes just walking from the back to the front of the house in a hurry would bring it on.

Bernard's doctor sent him for a *stress test*—an electrocardiogram taken while running on a treadmill or riding a stationary bicycle. His cardiogram showed changes as soon as the speed of the treadmill was increased. "I flunked the test," says Bernard.

Mary L. is a forty-five-year-old manager of a fashionable boutique in New York City. Her pressure-packed job in-

1

cludes frequent trips to Europe, spotting fashion trends and catering to a demanding clientele. She had always been in perfect health, but several months ago, she began to experience chest pain which she says felt "like a knot twisting in my chest." Sometimes the pain would shoot into her shoulder and neck, and sometimes it would be accompanied by a puffy kind of breathlessness that frightened her. Her electrocardiogram showed no irregularities, and Mary's physician prescribed medication which, so far, has relieved her pain.

Arthur P., seventy-five, had had chest discomfort for ten years. The pains, which he calls "pressure in the middle of my chest," began shortly after he retired from his job as a factory worker. He noticed them first during his daily four-mile walks on Ocean City's boardwalk. "Every few blocks I would get this bad pain, and I had to stop and rest for a few minutes. But when the pain went away, I kept on going as long as I could until it came again. Then I rested again."

Arthur's doctor gave him a tiny white tablet which he told him to place under his tongue whenever the pain came. "Now the pains hardly come at all," Arthur says. "I only use the medicine a few times a year."

Bernard, Mary and Arthur all suffer from angina pectoris, the symptoms of coronary artery disease. The condition, sometimes called *atherosclerosis,* is, simply, the buildup of fatty and fibrous material in the inner linings of arteries that carry blood to the heart muscle. When these deposits, also called lesions or plaque, become thick enough, they may partially or totally cut off blood flow and prevent oxygen from reaching the heart muscle.

At birth, everyone's arteries are smooth and open, but gradually fatty deposits accumulate in them. The process may begin in early childhood and, for years, may produce no symptoms—no chest pain, no tightness, no shortness of breath. Nothing. In fact, evidence shows that two-thirds of a coronary artery may be filled with fatty deposits without producing symptoms. Only when more than 70 percent of the channel is blocked does the patient begin to experience discomfort. Therefore, large numbers of people have coronary artery disease without being aware of it.

The condition is more prevalent in men than in women (at least until they reach menopause). An extensive study from the Montreal Heart Institute that looked at 401 women and 1,919 men with definite angina showed that young women begin with less obstruction in the coronary arteries than men and, even at age seventy, do not reach the same likelihood of having extensive disease.

And while it is generally true that the older one gets, the more likely he or she is to have coronary artery disease, an intriguing study from the pathology branch of the National Heart, Lung, and Blood Institute (NHLBI) in Bethesda, Maryland, reports that "if you reach age ninety, you don't need to worry as much about coronary heart disease."

Drs. William C. Roberts and Bruce F. Waller examined the hearts of twenty patients, ranging in age from ninety to one hundred three, who had died from various causes. They found that the coronary arteries look good after age ninety and that the chances of having much coronary disease after ninety appear to be relatively small. The oldest person in the study, a one hundred three-year-old woman, had coronary arteries that were "clean as a whistle," Dr. Roberts said.

When symptoms of the condition do appear, they are often the kind described by Arthur, Bernard and Mary. Other people with the condition may never experience symptoms but may suffer from heart failure (which eventually produces different symptoms, such as shortness of breath).

Still others have heart attacks *(myocardial infarctions)*, which can result in sudden death. Unlike the pain associated with angina, heart-attack pain is usually more severe, lasts longer and is not eased by rest. It has been described as "crushing" or "squeezing," and those who have experienced it often say they have had the feeling of impending death. Profuse sweating, shortness of breath, nausea and vomiting may be present.

Heart-attack pain, again unlike angina pain, often is manifested when a person is resting. It may even awaken him or her from sleep. But the cause is the same—an inadequate supply of blood to the heart. In heart attacks, the shortage is so great and lasts so long that a part of the heart muscle is destroyed. The seriousness of the attack and the degree of incapacitation it brings depend on how much heart-muscle tissue was destroyed during the time it was deprived of blood. For more than 50 percent of people with coronary artery disease, a heart attack is the first sign of trouble.

Patients who experience sudden death usually do so within two hours after their attack. It occurs because the heart attack has affected the rhythm of the heart—the delicate electrical system—to the extent that it can no longer support life.

Howard, a forty-five-year-old advertising account executive, was such a victim. He had never been ill, had regular annual checkups in which his doctor gave him a "clean bill of health" and had once-a-year electrocardiograms which showed no abnormalities. He left his home one crisp October morning to visit a client. Two hours later, he was dead. His autopsy report indicated that he had almost total blockages in three arteries of his heart. His friends and family could not understand why Howard had never experienced pain or discomfort.

"Atherosclerosis is a little strange," explains Dr. Horace MacVaugh, chief of the division of thoracic and cardiovascular surgery at Philadelphia's Lankenau Hospital. "It affects different areas of the body in different people at different rates. But there is good evidence that almost everyone has it."

In fact, autopsies of young men killed in Korea, about nineteen or twenty years old, found remarkably advanced coronary disease in many of them. More than 90 percent had evidence of the disease, not yet serious, but there was something there.

Some people go through life showing no signs of artery disease. Others exhibit symptoms ranging from *claudication* in the leg (pain in the leg vessels after walking certain distances) to heart problems.

The most common heart problem is angina pectoris. It is characterized most of the time by chest pain or tightness, which some people say feels like indigestion. Others have described it "like an elephant sitting on my chest" or "walking against the wind."

There may be pain in the jaw, teeth or earlobe and numbness or tingling in any or all parts of the arms. Angina pain rarely occurs directly over the heart.

The symptoms usually appear when the work of the heart is increased by exercise, stress or eating a big meal. But sometimes it happens even when a person is resting. It is a sign that the blood flow to the heart has been temporarily reduced, and it is the heart muscle's response to inadequate oxygen. The pain usually lasts from three to five minutes and is relieved by rest.

There are many people, however, who have atherosclerosis but, like Howard, do not have symptoms. In fact, at one time the New York Heart Association set up "functional classifications" for persons with the condition.

Functional Class I includes persons who have cardiac disease, but who do not experience limitations of their physical activity. Ordinary physical activity does not result in extreme fatigue, palpitations, shortness of breath or anginal pain.

Functional Class II consists of persons with cardiac disease which results in slight limits on physical activity. They are comfortable when resting, but ordinary physical activity can cause fatigue, palpitations, shortness of breath or angina.

Functional Class III. These are patients whose cardiac disease causes them marked limitation of physical activity. They are comfortable at rest, but mild physical exertion causes fatigue, palpitations, shortness of breath or angina.

Functional Class IV includes patients with cardiac disease who cannot engage in physical activity without discomfort. They may even feel discomfort at rest, and any physical activity increases it.

Physicians often classify their patients based on these categories.

No one knows for sure what causes atherosclerosis in the first place. But there seems to be no question that persons with a family history of the condition are at greater risk. The disorder probably is not inherited, but the susceptibility to it is thought to be genetic.

It is difficult to predict the percentage of the population that is genetically predisposed to coronary artery disease because so few people are able to trace their family medical history back through several generations. But the Utah Coronary Project, headed by Dr. Roger R. Williams, associate professor of internal medicine at the University of Utah Medical Center, is looking at a million Utah residents and their "roots," traced back four to six generations. The data is being matched via computer with confirmed deaths from heart disease, as shown by hospital data and state death records.

An analysis of 8,944 deaths from coronary disease indicates that "deaths from heart attacks are strongly familial if they occur at an early age—before sixty-five in men and before seventy in women," says Dr. Williams. "Men with early coronary death often had fathers with the same problem, and women who died early from heart disease often had mothers with the same disorder," Dr. Williams says. In addition, however, most hospital records of these people showed that they had two or three additional coronary risk factors, such as smoking, high blood pressure or high cholesterol.

The propensity toward heart disease was even traced to children. The Utah project found that high cholesterol levels were evident in about half of the offspring, including very young children, in affected branches of some families with a genetic predisposition to early coronary disease. In one study, a mother and her two sons had very high levels of cholesterol in their blood. The mother was alive at age seventy-two, but her sons died of heart attacks at ages thirty-two and forty-five. One brother, the one who died at thirty-two, was a cigarette smoker. The other did not smoke. Dr. Williams says that "this is a likely example of smoking potentiating a genetic predisposition to early coronary disease. It also illustrates the relative resistance of females to coronary disease."

Dr. Williams defines a "familial disposition" to the condition as existing for a man if two or more coronary deaths have occurred before age sixty-five among brothers, father, grandfathers and uncles. For women, two female coronary deaths before age seventy in the same group of relatives would suggest a genetic propensity toward heart disease.

Another study of 6,900 Cincinnati schoolchildren shows that families with histories of premature cardiovascular disease are more likely to have children with a high risk of developing the condition. The study, which was carried out over seven years, examined such risk factors as cholesterol and *triglyceride* levels in blood, high blood pressure, eating, drinking and smoking habits. It found that the children of men who died of heart attacks before they were fifty had higher than average levels of triglycerides and low-density *lipoproteins,* which have been found to increase the risk of heart disease.

Because genetic history is so critical, skillful family physicians should be certain to ask their patients probing questions about the health of parents and grandparents and to consider that heart problems may "run in the family."

However, as Dr. J. Willis Hurst, one of the country's leading cardiologists (he was cardiologist to the late President Lyndon Johnson), points out, many persons with a strong family history of the disease never have any sign of it, and, conversely, a person may be stricken with atherosclerosis even if there is no known trace of it in grandparents, parents or siblings. What, then, makes the difference?

Evidence is piling up that individual life-styles and certain physical risk factors count heavily.

In fact, the surge in recognizable heart disease since the early 1900s has been called by some "The Twentieth-Century Phenomenon," directly attributable to sweeping changes in life-style. Dr. John Farquhar of Stanford University, who has studied the history of heart disease, says that "it is likely that the incidence of heart attack in the forty-to-seventy age group was only a fifth as bad in 1910 as it is now." And Dr. Jeremiah Stamler of Northwestern University blames the twentieth-century life-style, characterized by affluence and stress, on the increased incidence of heart disease.

Some of the factors most often indicted are:

Smoking   Myriad studies verify that there is an undeniable association between smoking and premature coronary artery disease. Of the many toxic chemicals in cigarette smoke, carbon monoxide and nicotine appear to be the chief damagers of the cardiovascular system. Carbon monoxide interferes with the transportation of oxygen and the ability of heart tissues to use it effectively.

Nicotine is so lethal that if a person swallowed the amount contained in five cigarettes, he or she would die within a few minutes. According to Dr. Peter Kuo, chief of cardiology and professor of medicine at Rutgers Medical School, nicotine corrodes the smooth inner linings of vessel walls of the heart and stimulates the sympathetic nervous system to release adrenaline, which makes the heart beat faster and waste oxygen. Nicotine also blocks the liver's ability to dispose of blood fats after eating, thus leaving the fats to circulate through the blood and come to rest in arteries. As if this were not enough, the oxygen-carrying capacity of the red blood cells is compromised, thus depriving the heart muscle of oxygen. Smoking also increases blood pressure and contributes to an "irritable" heart muscle (one which produces erratic and irregular heartbeats).

Smokers of low-tar filter cigarettes gain no protection from the ravages of carbon monoxide. A heavy smoker, even if he uses only low-tar cigarettes, will inhale carbon monoxide levels eight times as high as levels considered safe in factories.

The average smoker doubles his chances of having a heart attack and of dying from it. A middle-aged man who smokes forty cigarettes a day dies from coronary disease at a rate more than ten times as high as a middle-aged man who does not smoke.

A recent French study, the Paris Prospective Study, found that a simple blood test can predict the risk of heart attack among middle-aged male smokers. The study included 7,206 Paris city workers and was conducted over six and a half years. It revealed that heavy smokers have high numbers of white blood cells, which are called *leuko-cytes*. The more leukocytes a person has, the greater are his or her chances of suffering a heart attack. These results confirmed an earlier study which found the white blood count to be an accurate predictor of heart-attack risk, but, unlike the earlier research, the Paris Prospective Study found that the measurement only applies to smokers who inhale. The relationship between smoking and blood count appeared when the men had more than 7,000 leukocytes per cubic millimeter of blood. Men who inhaled and had counts above 9,000 had nearly four times as many heart attacks as those whose levels were under 7,000.

Female smokers run the same risk as male smokers, and if they also use oral contraceptives, their risk of heart disease increases even more.

Smoking has been called "self-induced air pollution," and Dr. Kuo says that cigars and pipes are as damaging as cigarettes. People who convince themselves that low-tar cigarettes are "safe" are fooling no one. The only safe way, agree the experts, is to become an ex-smoker.

Hypertension (high blood pressure) Normal blood pressure for an adult may range from 120/80 to 140/90. The first number refers to the systolic pressure (the beat of the heart when it is contracting), and the lower number expresses the diastolic pressure (the pressure level in the arteries when the heart is resting). It used to be thought that diastolic pressure was the most critical, but a famous study conducted with the citizens of Framingham, Massachusetts, indicates that both systolic and diastolic pressure, when elevated, carry additional risk.

In fact, there is some evidence that systolic pressure may be a better predictor than diastolic pressure for most cardiovascular problems that are outgrowths of hypertension.

The study began in 1948 with a group of 5,209 men and women between the ages of thirty and sixty-two who were examined twice a year for twenty years. Eighty-five percent of the participants completed the study. At each examination, three blood-pressure measurements were taken (the first by a nurse and the others by a physician) in the left arm of each person while he or she was seated. The first reading taken by the physician was the one recorded for analysis. Isolated systolic hypertension (this means without elevated diastolic pressure) was defined as systolic pressure of 160 or more with diastolic pressure below 95.

The twenty-year follow-up showed that, of 445 men and 287 women who suffered from coronary heart disease, in all cases the percentage of persons with elevated systolic pressure exceeded the percentage with elevated diastolic pressure.

While some physicians feel that medication is not effective in treating systolic hypertension when diastolic pressure is normal, Dr. W.B. Kannel, former director of the Framingham study, does not agree. He says that experience in geriatric hospitals suggests that medication can reduce isolated systolic pressure in the majority of people with the condition.

High blood pressure makes the heart work harder and accelerates the process of atherosclerosis. A publication printed by the U.S. Department of Health and Human Services suggests that blood pressure which goes up slightly to 150/95—a level considered to be only mild elevation—increases the risk of heart attack two and a half times over that of a person with a pressure of 120/80.

Data from the Framingham study demonstrate that the risk for one type of stroke increases 30 percent for each 10 degree increase in blood pressure throughout the range of pressures.

Another study by the Veterans Administration documents the significant effect that blood-pressure control has on deaths from cardiovascular disease.

Almost 35 million people in the United States are estimated to have definite high blood pressure and need drug therapy. Another 25 million have borderline elevations of blood pressure and need, at the least, careful monitoring. Unfortunately, only 5 million of those with the condition are taking medication and achieving control of their condition.

No one knows what causes the condition, although studies indicate that some people are susceptible to it because of heredity. Persons whose parents had hypertension are at greater risk, and they may be most affected by overweight, stress, drinking or smoking. However, these factors will not cause hypertension in persons not prone to the ailment. And while the word "hypertense" conjures up an image of an anxious, frenzied executive type, the hypertensive patient may be tense or relaxed, aggressive or passive, active or lethargic.

Hypertension has often been thought of as an older person's disease, but there is increasing evidence that it may be prevalent in men and women under thirty-five, and even in teenagers and younger children. Findings of elevated blood pressure in children may be clues that serious hypertension will develop later.

Most of the time no specific cause can be found, and the patient is said to have "primary hypertension." However, there are a few conditions that may produce hypertension as a symptom, and prudent physicians will check for these where it seems warranted. For example, hypertension accompanied by swelling of the ankles and insufficient removal of waste products could indicate kidney disease. Palpitations, apprehension and an excess of the chemical substance—*catecholamines*—could, when accompanied by hypertension, mean that there is a tumor of the adrenal gland. But these conditions are rare, and more than 90 percent of the cases of hypertension occur for reasons unknown.

Until recently, persons with diastolic pressures between 90 and 104 were considered to be only mildly hypertensive, implying that their conditions should not cause concern. However, the results of a recent study conducted by the National Heart, Lung, and Blood Institute in the National Institutes of Health demonstrate that this is not the case.

In a seven-year program which included 14 communities and 10,000 people, it was shown that even people with mild hypertension, if aggressively but appropriately treated, have fewer deaths from all causes than people who receive routine care or no care at all.

The study worked this way: The 10,000 participants, all with sustained diastolic pressures of 90 or more, were divided into two groups. Five thousand were referred to traditional care, which meant that some were treated by their family physicians or other physicians and some received no treatment at all. The other 5,000 were closely followed at special clinics set up and operated at NIH. They received what has become known as *stepped care,* which means that the first step was simple treatment with *diuretics* (medication which increases salt loss from the body through the urine). If this did not work, another medication was added. Step three required the addition of a *vasodilator,* which opens up narrow vessels which could be contributing to the high blood pressure. If hypertension was still not reduced, step four introduced another drug.

"We found that the vast majority—80 to 85 percent—

was controlled either by a diuretic or by a diuretic and one additional drug," says Graham W. Ward, chief of the Institutes' Health Education Branch. "There were 17 percent fewer deaths in the group of patients who had received 'stepped care' than there were in the group that had received traditional care.

"We believe that our study has shown that persons with blood pressures of more than one hundred forty over ninety cannot be casually ignored," Ward says.

High blood pressure has been called "the silent killer" because it often produces no warning signals that it is present. That is why it is essential that every person, including children and teenagers, have blood-pressure measurements taken annually. The procedure is simple and painless; the doctor wraps a rubber device around the arm and inflates it as the blood pressure is read. (The device is called a *sphygmomanometer.*)

Today, blood-pressure machines can be found frequently in shopping malls, drugstores and banks. For a nominal fee (usually fifty cents), it is possible to obtain blood-pressure readings between visits to a physician. The doctor should be seen if a sustained rise in pressure is noticed.

Alcoholic binges   While some studies show that mild drinking, perhaps a drink with dinner each night, may help prevent heart disease, research from the Medical College of Wisconsin suggests that a drinking binge every now and then may be damaging to the heart.

"The crucial factor seems to be the difference between what a person usually drinks and the amount he or she drinks on these special occasions," says Dr. Harvey W. Gruchow, the epidemiologist who headed the study. The study found that men who drank three times their normal amount every so often (less than once a week) had 50 percent more heart blockage than those who drank only twice the normal amount. There is speculation that "binge" drinking may be harmful because it interferes with the formation of high-density lipoprotein cholesterol that scientists think may be beneficial to the heart.

Diabetes Diabetes, as evidenced by a trace or more of sugar in the urine or a measurement of glucose (sugar) of 120 milligrams or more in the blood, increases the risk of coronary disease. The risk of coronary artery disease is twice as great in diabetic men and three times as great in diabetic women as in persons who do not have the condition. Women, who usually have greater resistance to coronary artery disease than men, approach the same mortality rates from the disease when they are diabetic. Physicians can detect diabetes and prescribe drugs and diet to keep it under control.

Obesity Overweight itself is not thought to directly affect the heart, but it is linked with other risk factors, such as high blood pressure, cholesterol and blood sugar levels and, therefore, should be controlled.

The Framingham study found that the overweight person has a greater chance of developing angina than someone of normal weight. The chances increase as the weight rises. The same study reported a relationship between obesity and sudden death from heart attack. Persons who were more than 20 percent over their ideal weight had a chance of sudden death more than three times greater than their normal-weight counterparts.

Use of Oral Contraceptives A number of studies has confirmed that use of the birth-control pill has created hypertension in women who, before using the pill, had normal blood-pressure readings. Oral contraceptives have also been shown to raise the blood pressure, even within normal range, in almost all women who take them. Dr. W. B. Kannel, who directed the Framingham Heart Study, says that this "shift in the distribution of blood pressure has ominous long-term implications, because for each 10 mm Hg increment in pressure [in other words, a rise from 130 to 140 systolic], an estimated 30 percent increase in cardiovascular-disease incidence was noted in the Framingham Study."

Other studies have shown that oral contraceptives affect the *lipids* (fats) in the blood and that cholesterol—and especially triglyceride—levels can become elevated in women who use the pill.

Dr. Kannel warns that once women begin using the pill, they should be checked regularly for blood-pressure readings, blood lipids and glucose tolerance (sugar tolerance). If these characteristics develop or worsen, he believes birth-control pills should be discontinued. He is especially concerned with women who are hypertensive to start with, who have toxemia, who tend to gain weight at menstruation, who are overweight, who are diabetic or who are black (black women have greater tendency toward high blood pressure). He emphasizes that women who will not give up smoking should not be using oral contraceptives.

Stress   Anxiety and stress cause the "fight or flight" syndrome with which most people are familiar. The body's response to a fight with one's spouse, an argument with the boss or the death of a loved one often results in increased internal secretions that are controlled by areas in the brain. The symptoms are an increased heart rate, increased blood flow to the muscles and elevated blood pressure. It is a useful response that helps people meet a crisis; but when it is prolonged, it may contribute significantly to coronary artery disease.

For example, the cause of 90 percent of high blood pressure is not specifically known. It is thought that the "fight or flight" mechanism has a lot to do with it. People in rural areas generally have lower blood pressures than people who live at a feverish pace in busy cities. Examination time for students and tax time for accountants may send pressures soaring. Other studies show that major changes in one's life—moving to a new city, beginning a new job, a child leaving home, an ailing parent—are associated with increased risk of coronary artery disease. While most people can adapt to some change, many changes in life during a short period, or chronic "overload," can be dangerous.

But Dr. Herbert Benson, a Harvard professor and director of the division of behavioral medicine at Beth Israel Hospital in Boston, says that while stress is unavoidable, people can learn to control the way their bodies respond to it. There are techniques (discussed in Chapter 7) through which one can decrease the activity of the sympathetic nervous system, which, if fast-paced, can propel one on the road to heart disease.

Personality and Behavior Pattern   Persons identified as having "Type A" behavior are shown to be at greater risk of coronary heart disease. Type A's are characterized by being competitive, ambitious, unable to relax, more hostile and always feeling as though there is not enough time to accomplish everything he or she would like.

The concept was introduced and intensively studied by Drs. Meyer Friedman and Ray Rosenman, two California cardiologists who say that partial credit for the finding must go to the woman who was president of San Francisco's Junior League in the mid-1950s.

"We were testing the theory that women are protected from heart disease because they ate foods lower in fat and

cholesterol than men," says Dr. Friedman. Members of
the Junior League agreed to cooperate in the test by
filling in and having their husbands fill in, for a two-week
period, a diary of everything that they ate (without changing their diets from what they ate normally) during that
time.

But before the experiment started, the president of the
Junior League warned, "You'll find that we are eating
exactly the same way our husbands are. It is the stress on
Montgomery Street [San Francisco's business district]
that is killing them. My husband has to have two martinis
when he comes home at night just to unhinge his jaw."

The woman was correct. The diaries revealed no differences between the men and women in their eating habits.
But there was a difference in the way they met to learn
the doctors' findings.

"We had a meeting, scheduled for two P.M., to which
only the women were invited," Dr. Friedman recalls.
"Some of the women arrived a little after two, some at
two-fifteen, and some meandered in at two-thirty. It
wasn't until two forty-five that we could begin the meeting. Some of the women wore watches, but many of them
[the watches] weren't working. And at about twenty minutes into the meeting, we asked the women if they knew
where the clock was on the wall. They didn't.

"But the next week, when we invited the men to a
similar meeting, they arrived promptly at two," Dr.
Friedman said. "They all had watches and, after about
twenty minutes, began looking at them impatiently.
When we asked them where the clock was, almost all of
them knew."

Stimulated by these findings, the doctors contacted
three companies and sent them questionnaires to distrib-
ute among their employees. "Which factors do you think
are responsible for heart attacks?" the questionnaire

asked. There were ten choices. Seventy-five percent of the respondents checked "stress" and "the pressure of deadlines." The doctors then distributed the same questionnaires to ninety physicians. The results were the same. Seventy-five percent thought that it was meeting deadlines, stress and excessively competitive activity that caused heart disease.

"If we had been more alert, we may have considered more carefully a remark made to us before all of these experiments," says Dr. Friedman. "We had called in an upholsterer to fix the seats on our office chairs. Midway through, he asked us what kind of practice we had, because he noticed that the upholstery was worn away only on the front edge of the seat, indicating that our patients were not sitting back, relaxed, in their chairs."

Results of the experiments and recall of the upholsterer's remark stimulated the doctors' investigation into the behavior of their heart patients. What they found was a pattern of behavior exhibited by persons with certain personalities when confronted by challenge.

Typically, this behavior pattern, which they labeled Type A, involves a chronic and excessive struggle to obtain an unlimited number of things from the environment in the shortest possible time and, if necessary, against formidable opposition. Type A people generally speak quickly in voices that frequently shift pitch; they finish other people's sentences because they grow impatient, even irritable, waiting for the person to complete his thought; they will easily show anger and hostility (sometimes through the use of profanities), and they may show annoyance by clenching their fists or pounding on a table to make a point.

The mechanism through which Type A behavior leads to heart disease, says Dr. Friedman, is an increase in the production of a neuro-hormone put out by the *autonomic nervous system,* the system that governs involuntary functions. Anxiety and stress cause an increase in the production of the hormone that, in turn, causes cholesterol levels to rise, hastens the clotting time of blood and constricts blood vessels that supply blood to the heart.

Today, Type A behavior is recognized as an established factor in coronary artery disease. The National Heart, Lung, and Blood Institute issued a statement saying, "The review panel [of the Institute] accepts the available body of scientific evidence as demonstrating that Type A behavior is associated with an increased risk of clinically apparent coronary disease in employed, middle-aged United States citizens. The increased risk is over and above that imposed by age, systolic blood pressure, serum cholesterol and smoking and appears to be of the same order of magnitude as the relative risk associated with any of these other factors." The findings of Drs. Friedman and Rosenman have been widely confirmed by others in this country, Canada and Europe.

Exercise.   Some studies suggest that sedentary living may contribute to coronary artery disease and, conversely, that appropriate physical activity may protect against the condition and improve the likelihood of survival from a coronary attack. A theory is that exercise reduces stress because it lowers the levels of hormones that increase the heart rate and blood pressure. It also helps in keeping weight under control and in increasing a person's ability to dissolve blood clots.

However, Dr. Michael Ellis DeBakey, one of the world's most famous heart surgeons, says that while there is some evidence that a high degree of physical activity will prevent heart attacks and atherosclerosis, this has not been proven in a scientifically controlled experiment.

Others, however, such as Dr. Thomas F. Santilli, medical director of the Human Performance Laboratory at Philadelphia's Holy Redeemer Hospital, firmly believe that a sedentary person increases his chances of becoming a coronary victim.

An experiment on young athletes who spent twenty days in bed showed that their intake of oxygen was reduced by at least 25 percent and that the pumping capacity of the heart was similarly decreased.

A study recently reported in *Lancet* which followed more than 17,000 persons over a ten-year period found that those who were active had less coronary disease than those who were sedentary. The difference was three times less—6.9 percent incidence of coronary disease in sedentary persons compared to 3 percent in those who were active. No matter which other risk factors a person had (hypertension, smoking, and so on), lack of vigorous exercise was considered an independent risk factor for coronary disease.

And the President's Council on Physical Fitness maintains that persons who do not exercise at least a half-hour a day may be less fit physically than is optimally desirable. And that half-hour of exercise should be of the nature that will increase heartbeat rate and elevate blood pressure. Exercise, many believe, will make the heart work better because it will be able to pump blood with less effort. Also, developing a capacity for increased exercise tolerance without tiring can be translated into management of physical or emotional crises without straining the heart or elevating the blood pressure.

On the other hand, Dr. William B. Kannel, professor of medicine at Boston University and former director of the Framingham Heart Study (the largest of its kind), says that exercise is only valuable if it is used as part of a total approach in protecting the heart, which includes not smoking, reducing high blood pressure and eating properly. And San Francisco's Dr. Friedman says that there is no scientific evidence to show that exercise prevents heart disease. He feels, in fact, that persons who have had heart attacks should limit strenuous exercise. They should not jog, run or play handball or racketball. "When you stress a mechanism beyond its capacity, any defect will show," he says. Dr. Friedman says that a study on sudden death, in which he participated, showed that 50 percent of those deaths were immediately preceded by severe or moderate exercise.

Diet and Cholesterol   Eating "properly" means different things to different people, and the battle over the kind of diet that increases the odds of becoming a heart patient still simmers. It is generally felt that a diet high in salt, especially for persons who tend to be hypertensive, is damaging. Salt is often responsible for the body's retention of fluid, which strains the heart's pumping mechanism. It does this by adding extra pressure to the vessel wall and contributes to high blood pressure.

But the biggest controversy centers around cholesterol, a fatty substance (called a lipid) which is found in all living tissues. The body gets cholesterol in two ways: it manufactures its own; and it accumulates it through ingesting cholesterol-rich foods that are the mainstay of the diet of many Americans.

Most scientists agree that a person with a blood cholesterol level of 250 or more runs more than double the heart-attack risk than that of a person with a level below 194. And Nathan Pritikin, whose low-cholesterol diet is followed by a growing number of dedicated believers, says, "It is more important to know your cholesterol level than it is to know how many dollars are in your bank account." He advocates a cholesterol level of no more than 160.

Actually, the first admonition to lower body cholesterol probably can be found in the Bible. There, God instructs Moses to tell the children of Israel not to eat fat from oxen, sheep and goats. Since that time, warnings about the intake of cholesterol have come from the American Heart Association, the Senate Select Committee on Nutrition and Human Needs, the Departments of Agriculture and Health and Human Services. The architects of the famous Framingham study indict high cholesterol as one of the most potent precursors of heart disease.

High cholesterol content is found in many favorite foods: butter; eggs; ice cream; milk; cream; and marbleized, juicy steaks. Persons whose diets are rich in those foods are likely to be increasing their chances of suffering with clogged arteries that may lead to atherosclerosis, with its accompanying symptoms, such as angina.

The millions of Americans who enjoy those foods found temporary solace in a report issued by the Food and Nutrition Board of the National Academy of Sciences (a quasi-official Supreme Court in science), claiming that lowering intake of the "demon cholesterol" will probably not lower blood cholesterol in healthy individuals, will not prevent heart attacks and will not help people live longer with plaque-free arteries.

However, before people all over America saturated themselves on sizzling steaks and frothy soufflés, the study was soundly criticized as being "biased" and "scientifically unsound." Two key members of the panel were accused of lack of objectivity because they were paid consultants to food producers whose products would be affected by the study. Their clients, who provided approximately 10 percent of their income, included egg, dairy and other food interests, and it is their products that are rich in cholesterol and which have been linked to the instigation of atherosclerosis. Two other panel members have had research grants from the egg industry.

"The nutrition board was wrong when it concluded that it is scientifically unsound to recommend diets low in fat and cholesterol to prevent heart disease," declared the National Academy of Science's consumer panel. "Frankly, in a society which is being ravaged by coronary heart disease, I consider it irresponsible for someone to say, 'Go out and enjoy and eat anything you want,' " said Dr. William Castelli, director of the federal government's heart-disease study project in Framingham, Massachusetts. "This is no time to pour gas on the fire."

"There is a consensus among health experts that Americans should cut down on fat and cholesterol to reduce the risk of heart disease," echoed Dr. Kent Peterson, former executive vice-president of the American College of Preventive Medicine.

And a long-range study, published in the *New England Journal of Medicine*, reaffirmed that too much cholesterol and fat is, indeed, injurious. The study involved 1,900 male employees of Chicago's Western Electric Company and confirmed that middle-aged men whose diets are heavy in those substances suffer 30 percent more heart attacks than their counterparts who follow a diet lower in fats and cholesterol.

Each man's dietary habits were recorded, and they were given a physical examination. Their wives were questioned about the kind of food eaten in their homes. Food prepared in the company cafeteria and nearby restaurants was scrutinized. A year later, the men were examined again and classified into one of three groups, depending on how much fat and cholesterol they consumed. The researchers, headed by Dr. Richard Shekelle, a specialist in preventive medicine at Chicago's Rush-Presbyterian-St. Luke's Medical Center, found that initially, the cholesterol levels in the blood reflected the degree of fat and cholesterol consumption. A year later, the men who had lowered their intake of rich foods had less cholesterol in their blood. After nineteen years, the men who had eaten the most cholesterol had the most fatal heart attacks.

Cholesterol, however, is not the only culprit. The level of triglycerides (another lipid) in the blood is also considered by some to be critical. A high level would be a silent forewarner that the arteries of the heart are clogging. Foods which supply triglycerides are carbohydrates, such as those found in starches, sugars and some fresh fruit. Normal triglyceride levels range from 50 to 200, and it is prudent, many physicians believe, to maintain them within those boundaries. Triglyceride levels can be determined through simple blood tests.

In connection with cholesterol and triglycerides, the terms "high-density lipoproteins" (HDL) and "low-density lipoproteins" (LDL) are often used by doctors, but few patients understand what they mean or what their significance may be.

Low-density lipoproteins, which can be measured through blood tests, are composed of approximately 25 percent protein and 75 percent lipid (most of which is cholesterol). A high level of low-density lipoproteins is considered unhealthy. In fact, according to a report issued by the National Heart, Lung, and Blood Institute and the National Institutes of Health, persons with strikingly elevated low-density lipoproteins (a familial condition) frequently develop severe coronary disease by the time they are fifteen years old.

The Center for Inherited Diseases at the University of Washington in Seattle is studying excessive levels of blood fats and their causes. The center, headed by Dr. Arno Motulsky, has confirmed that a condition called *familial hypercholesterolemia* runs in families. The disease is caused by a single gene that alters the binding of low-density lipoprotein (LDL) by a specific site on a cell, called a receptor. Normally, a cell can capture LDL, the "bad" lipoprotein, and keep it from accumulating in the body. But a defective receptor permits the LDL to accumulate, thus setting the stage for atherosclerosis. This condition occurs in about one in five hundred individuals in the general population, but in Seattle it was found in 5 percent of males who had had a heart attack at age sixty or younger. There is a specific laboratory test for familial hypercholesterolemia, Dr. Motulsky says, but it is costly and complex, and not adaptive to routine laboratory use. More feasible tests are being investigated.

High-density lipoproteins are another story. They consist of approximately 50 percent protein and 50 percent lipid and are often called "the good cholesterol." Dr. Robert Levy, former director of the National Heart, Lung, and Blood Institute in Bethesda, following studies conducted at ten medical research centers, says that higher levels of "this good cholesterol are associated with a reduced risk of heart attack." Curiously, the "good cholesterol" sometimes increases after one or two drinks of alcohol a day.

Dr. Levy is not certain exactly how this "good" substance works in the body, but he says that studies of more than 10,000 people revealed that those with large amounts of high-density lipoproteins were far less likely to contract atherosclerosis and its resulting conditions, particularly heart disease.

The only substance known to be positively related to this "good cholesterol" is niacin—a B vitamin found in meats, enriched cereals, potatoes, nuts and yeast—when ingested in high doses.

But for reasons not yet determined, life-style and education appear to influence the amount of the substance in the blood. Men and women who have completed one or more years of college have higher levels of high-density lipoprotein than those with fewer years of education, according to a report from the Lipid Research Clinics Program in the University of North Carolina at Chapel Hill.

Levels of HDL are also higher in long-distance runners and joggers as well as in moderate consumers of alcohol. They are lower in cigarette smokers and persons who are 20 percent or more over the acceptable weight for their height, age and body build.

The Chapel Hill study was conducted on 2,182 white women and 2,368 white men at nine institutions throughout the country. Those who participated were divided into two age groups: twenty to thirty-nine, and forty to fifty-nine.

The findings suggested that men and women with more years of formal education may be more aware of the importance of good personal health habits, that they may learn more about how to protect themselves from problems such as heart attacks, that they may eat more sensibly, smoke less and see to it that they get more exercise.

The consensus is that life-style—which includes such factors as blood pressure, cholesterol and triglyceride levels—smoking habits, glucose tolerance, sex, age, exercise habits and personality type all count heavily in determining who will and who will not eventually become victims of heart disease. The effects of elevated blood pressure, high cholesterol and smoking are approximately the same.

The American Heart Association publishes a *Coronary Risk Handbook* which charts the probability of developing heart disease based on those factors. For instance, a fifty-five-year-old man who does not smoke, has a healthy heart muscle, is not diabetic, has a cholesterol level of 185 and a systolic blood pressure of 180 has a 9.0 chance (out of 100) of developing coronary artery disease in the next six years. The same man with a cholesterol level of 335 increases the odds to 18.8.

A woman of the same age and description, with a cholesterol level of 185 and systolic blood pressure of 180, has a 3.8 chance of becoming a coronary patient in the next half-dozen years. But if her cholesterol level increases to 335, her risk increases to 9.4.

However, despite the linkage between the risk factors and the disease, there are people who seem to be certain candidates but who never show signs of the condition. And there are others whose demographics would put them in the category of "unlikely victims," yet they develop severe angina or may even have a heart attack.

How much do we know about what makes the difference? Dr. Gerald Lemole, chairman of the department of surgery at Deborah Heart and Lung Center in Browns Mills, New Jersey, has a theory. He conjectures that the lymphatic systems in some people are just more efficient than in others. The lymphatic system contains the fluid that bathes each cell of the body and clears out poisons, toxins, bacteria and other harmful elements. While the effectiveness of the lymph system in an individual probably has a lot to do with genetics, Dr. Lemole feels it can be influenced by exercise and a positive mental attitude that can often result from meditation, relaxing activities or even a vacation. Conversely, stress and lack of exercise can compromise the ability of the lymphatic system to protect the body against atherosclerosis.

Dr. William B. Kannel, famous for the Framingham Study, has said that there is a simple test that can predict—as accurately as blood cholesterol, levels of high-density lipoprotein, insulin level, blood pressure or age

—a person at high risk of cardiovascular disease. It is a breathing test, taken with an instrument called a *spirometer*, through which physicians can measure the amount of air a person can hold in his or her lungs and the force with which it can be expelled. If a person's capacity to hold air in his lungs and to expel it decreases, it is a sign that he is not as fit as he should be, says Dr. Kannel. He says that it is a warning that the person should begin looking at his blood pressure, diet, lack of exercise and smoking habits in order to increase the efficiency of his body. Women who are at high risk of heart disease can expel less than two liters of air, Dr. Kannel explains, while low-risk women can expel four liters (almost five quarts).

Philadelphia's Dr. Santilli says, "I firmly believe that the problem of coronary artery disease as it now exists has no single answer. And we do not have the luxury of eternity as far as answers are concerned. The best approach is to accept and put into operation those principles which seem to be protective, and to be responsive to change when newer evidence requiring different action does appear."

While there are many ways an individual can prevent the development of coronary heart disease, there was not, until recently, a great deal physicians were able to do to give patients long-term relief from the pain of angina. Standard treatment has been, and in some cases still is, the use of *nitroglycerin* as a stopgap measure. Patients with angina carried tiny white pills and placed one under the tongue whenever the uncomfortable tight, strangling sensation started. Such patients were advised to change their life-styles—to eliminate smoking, slow down their pace, take more frequent vacations, switch to a lower-pressure job. But since the condition is usually progressive, people who suffered severe discomfort were often forced to embrace a sedentary way of life, giving up many previous activities and pleasures.

It was no wonder, then, that the advent of the coronary artery bypass in the late 1960s found a multitude of heart patients willing, even eager, to go under the knife.

2 WHAT IS THE BYPASS OPERATION, AND WHY IS IT SO CONTROVERSIAL?

Larry R., fifty-two, is a Chicago attorney with an impressive list of big-name clients. He was a whiz in the courtroom, traveled to Egypt and Singapore and Marseilles on behalf of his clients and was known as the city's most eligible bachelor.

That was twenty-two years ago, when Larry was thirty and facing what he thought was going to be a sparkling future. But without warning, his neat little universe began to crumble around him. One misty March morning in 1959, he was stricken by a severe pain in his chest that almost knocked him over.

"I'll never forget that first time," Larry says. "I was sure I was having a heart attack. I was in the courtroom, trying a case. It was a case about a man with a large estate, who had died and left his money to a woman who was a good friend. He specifically excluded from his will all members of his family and directed that some of his money go to a children's charity fund. His family protested that he had been mentally unfit when he made his will, that he had been influenced and coerced. I knew the man who had died, and I believed, without question, that he knew exactly what he was doing. But there was a history of some emotional instability in his life, and he had been in group therapy for a while.

31

"Anyway, I was getting very passionate about this whole thing, and during the trial, I got more than a little excited. Suddenly this incredible pain came, right in the center of my chest, and it took my breath away. It came with no warning, and I had to stop for a couple of minutes. But amazingly enough, it went away when I sat down, and I was able to go on with the case. I won, too," he says, smiling.

Unfortunately, that was only the beginning of what turned out to be a sixteen-year-long nightmare. Larry's pains came more often and grew progressively worse. The medication his doctor gave him didn't help. Neither did giving up smoking. Or drinking. Or sex.

"Gradually, I had to stop doing almost everything," Larry remembers. "If I went to a restaurant and had a terrific dinner, I would suffer later. If I became emotional over a client, I would get pain. If I dated a woman and we had an argument, there came the pains again.

"It seemed as though I wouldn't be able to do anything except sit in a rocking chair for the rest of my life. I guess I became a hypochondriac. I tiptoed through my life as though I were walking on jagged glass. There was nothing I felt comfortable doing. I would even prescreen movies and television shows to make sure there was nothing in them that would agitate me. I stopped reading the bad news in the newspaper. I read books about subjects that had no interest for me—things like gardening—because I thought the tranquility might be good.

"Night after night, I closeted myself in my bedroom, wondering, 'What did I ever do to deserve this?'

"Years later, when I began to hear about an operation that might help the condition, I didn't want to explore it. I was certain that the strain of any operation would surely kill me. My doctor knew how I felt, so he didn't push it either.

"But then one of my sister's friends, a man twenty years older than I but with similar symptoms, had surgery that turned him into a new person. He was able to go back to work (which he hadn't done for four years); he could dance with his wife again. He even played tennis.

"So I decided to talk to him about it. Then I talked to my doctor about it. Then I thought about it some more. But I had so many questions. It was the most difficult decision I had ever had to make."

The operation that Larry had to ponder was a new one at the time: coronary bypass surgery. It was performed most often to relieve just the kind of pain that Larry had.

An early attempt to operate on the heart to relieve the symptoms of atherosclerosis was made by a Canadian physician, Arthur Vineberg, in 1946, but results of his procedure were unpredictable and often unsatisfactory. However, the operation (known medically as *myocardial revascularization*) in wide use today was developed a little more than a decade ago by Dr. R. Favaloro at the Cleveland Clinic (Dr. Favaloro is now chief of thoracic and cardiovascular surgery at the Guemes' Foundation in Buenos Aires, Argentina) and Dr. W. Dudley Johnson, associate clinical professor of surgery at the departent of thoracic-cardiovascular surgery at the Medical College of Wisconsin. (There is, however, a report in the medical literature, published by Drs. H. Edward Garrett, Edward W. Dennis and Michael E. DeBakey, of a successful coronary bypass operation at the Baylor College of Medicine in November 1964 on a forty-two-year-old truck driver. The report was not published until 1973 after arteriography showed that the graft inserted was still open.)

The operation involves bypassing the blocked portions of any or all of the three major coronary arteries (the arteries which carry blood to the heart muscle itself)—the left main, the right or the circumflex—and often some of

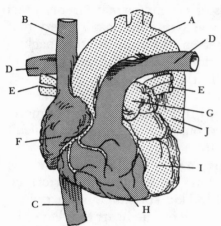

HEART: EXTERIOR VIEW
A - AORTIC ARCH
B - SUPERIOR VENA CAVA
C - INFERIOR VENA CAVA
D - PULMONARY ARTERY
E - PULMONARY VEIN
F - RIGHT ATRIUM
G - LEFT ATRIUM
H - RIGHT VENTRICLE
I - LEFT VENTRICLE
J - AORTA

HEART: CROSS-SECTION
A - SUPERIOR VENA CAVA
    (FROM HEAD AND ARMS)
B - INFERIOR VENA CAVA
C - RIGHT ATRIUM
D - LEFT ATRIUM
E - RIGHT VENTRICLE
F - LEFT VENTRICLE
G - PULMONARY ARTERY
H - PULMONARY VEIN
I - AORTIC ARCH
    (TO HEAD AND ARMS)
J - AORTA
K - VENTRICULAR SEPTUM
L - ENDOCARDIUM
M - MYOCARDIUM
N - EPICARDIUM
O - PERICARDIUM
P - TRICUSPID VALVE
Q - MITRAL VALVE
R - PULMONARY VALVE
S - AORTIC VALVE

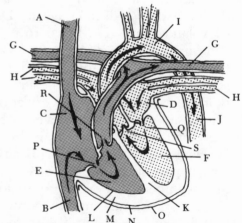

Courtesy of The National Heart, Lung, and Blood Institute.

their subsidiary branches with *saphenous veins.* These are the same veins that are stripped from a patient's legs to correct varicosity, and they are removed at the same time the bypass operation is performed. In some cases, the bypass is accomplished through using an internal mammary artery—one of the many arteries carrying blood to the chest wall—instead of the leg vein.

Certain clogged arteries are more worrisome than others. To understand why, it is critical to know the anatomy of the heart and how it works.

The heart, a hollow, muscular organ, is situated in the center of the chest, a little to the left. It is protected by the sternum (the breastbone) and the rib cage. The heart's job is to pump blood, which is rich in oxygen and other nutrients, to all parts of the body.

The blood pumps through the body's arterial-vascular system, which means that arteries (including the aorta, the largest artery) carry blood away from the heart to cells throughout the body, and veins pick up blood from those cells and return the blood to the heart. The blood that returns, however, contains waste products, including carbon dioxide.

There are four chambers in the heart. The two upper chambers, or atria, receive the blood that is carried to them by the veins. The ventricles, or two lower chambers, pump blood out of the heart. Four valves direct the blood flow, and a septum (wall) divides the heart into a right side and a left side. It is the right side of the heart that receives blood from the body and pumps it to the lungs. The lungs cleanse the blood of waste products (carbon dioxide) and provide it with a fresh supply of oxygen.

The left side of the heart receives the recycled blood from the lungs and pumps it into the *aorta.* The arterial system of the heart originates from the aorta (the main artery of the body), which supplies blood through the arterial branches to the entire body. And then there are the left and right coronary arteries, each of which divides into smaller branches that are responsible for nourishing all areas of the heart itself.

The first portion of the left coronary artery is called the left main artery. The left main divides into branches—the left anterior descending (called LAD) and the circumflex. The LAD provides nourishment to the front of the heart muscle, and the circumflex supplies blood to the back of the heart. The right coronary artery supplies blood to the right side of the heart and has branches which reach to the rear of the heart.

The average adult has about ten pints of blood circulating through the body all the time. Two and a half ounces of blood are squeezed out or ejected by the heart with each beat. Each minute, while a person is at rest, the heart pumps four to five quarts of blood through the body. When a person is exercising or is under stress, this can increase to twenty quarts a minute. To do its job effectively, the heart muscle must be nourished from its own blood supply, which it receives from the network of coronary arteries.

When this network is functioning well, it provides the heart muscle with a half a pint of blood a minute, at rest, and up to a quart of blood a minute with exercise.

When atherosclerosis has not progressed to more than 50 percent, most people will have no symptoms; but when it exceeds 50 percent, an inadequate supply of blood will be furnished to the heart when the person is exercising or stressed. If the blockages get to be 85 or 90 percent, a person is likely to feel discomfort even at rest, because occlusions this severe prevent blood from getting through even when there is no activity. Often the heart compensates by creating small collateral channels from another artery. But in many cases this does not happen, or the created channels are inadequate, and a portion of the heart muscle, starved by a lack of oxygen-rich blood, will die. This is known as a heart attack.

Almost half of all middle-aged men with coronary artery disease have a heart attack as their first sign. But about 25 percent experience angina as a warning that their arteries are clogged.

Most people who undergo surgery for clogged arteries are bypassed with veins from their legs. However, the mammary artery is sometimes considered to be superior. In fact, the Cleveland Clinic, one of the nation's leading centers for bypass surgery, uses it in 32 percent of its cases.

"The mammary artery has a ten to fifteen percent higher patency rate than saphenous vein grafts (grafts made with the mammary artery tend to stay open longer than those done with saphenous veins) but it is not nearly as versatile an operation in that the left mammary artery can reach easily only to the anterior coronary artery," says Dr. Loop. "Grafting the mammary artery to the coronary artery is technically more difficult than a vein graft. Also, it takes slightly longer to produce a mammary-artery graft because of the time required to mobilize the artery from the chest wall," Dr. Loop says.

Dr. Favaloro, one of the originators of the bypass operation, agrees. "Operations with the internal mammary artery are much more difficult to perform and must be done precisely to attain good results."

Everyone has two mammary arteries, one on either side of the breastbone. Dr. Loop says that they are "superb conduits" and can be used on virtually everybody except those patients who have a very large coronary artery, or those who have a very thick heart muscle because of hypertension or disease that involves the heart valves.

"We use it in about thirty to thirty-five percent of our

cases, and we have done more than eight thousand of these operations," he says.

Ten years of experience using the internal mammary artery was recounted by Dr. Jack C. Manley of St. Luke's Hospital in Milwaukee, at a 1981 meeting of the American Academy of Cardiologists. Dr. Manley said that for 5,922 internal-mammary-artery bypass grafts performed the incidence of surgical mortality, complication rate, postoperative exercise stress test, relief of angina and eight-year survival rates are comparable to results achieved in patients who received saphenous vein grafts. *Angiography* from one to eight years later revealed high patency rate (92 percent) in patients with the internal-mammary-artery graft. Dr. Manley and his colleagues, in an abstract which appeared in the *American Journal of Cardiology*, conclude that, "In view of higher patency rates, this conduit is preferable alone or in combination with saphenous-vein bypass graft."

In addition to the increased chances of the graft made with the mammary artery remaining open, there are other benefits. Its size correlates more closely than does the size of the leg vein with the smaller coronary arteries. "This accounts for the higher patency rate," Dr. Loop explains, "and is particularly good for people who have failed grafts [grafts that did not remain open and resulted in renewed pain for the patient] to the anterior descending coronary artery. There seems to be less appearance of atherosclerosis in the conduit [the graft] when it is a mammary artery than when it is a vein, over a period of years."

Using the mammary artery has the advantage of avoiding an incision in the leg to remove the saphenous vein. Some patients, especially women, object to the scar that such a procedure produces. More important, use of the mammary artery eliminates the discomfort of another incision. In fact, many people who have had bypass surgery where the saphenous vein has been used have complained that they were more bothered by leg pain than chest pain.

Other practitioners do not agree that the mammary artery is especially advantageous, but Dr. Loop insists that his hospital is looking at results over a long period and that a lot of information has been accumulated to show that the mammary artery is at least as good as, and possibly better than, veins from the leg, because they stay open longer.

"If you look at vein grafts to the anterior descending coronary artery as compared with mammary-artery grafts, the mammary artery has a ten percent higher patency in our institution. Some people may challenge this, but they are probably looking at very early results [results soon after surgery]. When you get out beyond a year after the surgery, the mammary artery has a decided advantage."

Dr. Loop does not use mammary-artery grafts on older people, on people with very severe angina, in instances where the mammary artery itself may be diseased or, most important, where there is a large coronary vessel in a heart that has *left ventricular hypertrophy* (thickening of the left ventricle muscle because of an increased pressure load on the ventricle. A possible cause could be hypertension). These are usually people with a long history of hypertension or disease of the valves of the heart.

In any case, one end of the graft vessel is sewn to the coronary artery below the area of blockage, and the other is attached to the aorta, the main artery. In this way, oxygen-rich blood is taken directly from the aorta, bypasses the obstruction and flows through the graft to nourish the heart muscle.

It is a process of rerouting, something like a highway underpass or overpass that permits a driver to avoid

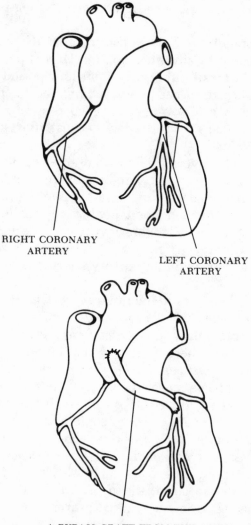

RIGHT CORONARY
ARTERY

LEFT CORONARY
ARTERY

A BYPASS GRAFT FROM THE AORTA
TO ONE OF THE CORONARY ARTERIES

Courtesy of The National Heart, Lung, and Blood Institute.

clogged city streets. Because the blood supply flows freely once more, the heart muscle receives more of it and is able to pump more effectively. The improvement, if all goes well, is immediate and begins even before the patient leaves the operating room.

The operation became feasible when the heart-lung machine was perfected. This is a space-age-looking device that breathes for the patient while he or she is on the operating table. It permits the surgeon to work for the several hours that bypass operations take on a heart that is still, not pumping, because a machine is doing it instead.

While the heart-lung machine has been in active use only since the late 1960s, it was the dream of a Philadelphia doctor, John G. Gibbon, who recognized that long operations to correct heart defects could be accomplished only if the heart were "still" for the period of time during which the surgeon performed his handicraft.

During that time, something had to take over the most important function of the lungs and heart—taking venous blood from the patient, removing carbon dioxide from it, infusing it with oxygen and pumping the blood back through the body. If this process is interrupted, even for a few minutes, the brain will die.

Dr. Gibbon's use of a device that would literally become the patient's lungs and heart during surgery failed in two patients, and he became disenchanted with the concept. Still, he and his wife, who was a laboratory technician, experimented with cats and dogs, opening and suturing their hearts while they were "on bypass" (the expression used by surgeons to describe the part of the procedure during which the heart-lung machine takes over the patient's breathing), then determining whether their normal functioning could resume.

In 1953, Dr. Gibbon began to use the procedure on human beings. There was one success, a baby whose half-hour operation was performed while she was "on bypass," and who lived with her heart defect corrected. But three other patients died, and Dr. Gibbon abandoned his project. It was up to other physicians all over the world to continue perfecting the machine. Early models were crude, even though they worked. But as the heart-lung machine became more refined and more sophisticated, it revolutionized the treatment of heart disease.

In the beginning, the operation was considered by patients to be a "miracle"; an answer to their prayers; an escape at last from the pain, discomfort and restricted life-styles they had been forced to embrace. Physicians were equally as enthusiastic about being able to offer their distressed patients an alternative that could bring them relief.

Each year, since 1967, more heart patients have opted for the operation. By 1980, more than 500,000 patients had undergone it. In many of the leading medical centers, there are long waiting lists; patients must be prepared, except in emergencies, to stand by sometimes for months for their place on the operating table. There is every indication that the numbers of people desiring the surgery will continue to increase. The Deborah Heart and Lung Center in Browns Mills, New Jersey, for instance, which performed 750 open-heart operations in 1976 and 850 in 1978, is projecting 1,600 in 1985. Dr. Denton Arthur Cooley, surgeon-in-chief of the Texas Heart Institute in Houston and one of the leading authorities in the field, and his team performed 2,800 bypass operations in 1980 and expects that number to increase. Patients count on the surgery to relieve their pain, cure their disease and prolong their lives.

However, in the past few years, there have been rumblings of discontent within medical circles. There have been claims that patients have been misled about what the operation can accomplish and, therefore, go into surgery with unrealistic expectations. Some physicians are not convinced that the surgery benefits patients more than meticulous management with medicine and drugs.

They talk (usually off the record) about grafts that do not remain open, the incidence of surgically induced heart attacks (that the patient may sometimes be unaware of) and the need for second and third operations.

They grumble about the widespread use of an operation before its risks and benefits were clearly defined, and of "incompetent surgeons" who have seen a good thing and have gotten on the bandwagon.

While the battle is being fought primarily in the medical world, inklings of it have trickled out to a more sophisticated, more demanding public, a public which no longer sees the "Physician as God," but which is questioning doctors' decisions and insisting on participating in its own health care.

Today, the men and women who are considering bypass surgery are asking their doctors more questions. After all, the operation, except in a small percentage of cases, is an elective one, and it is the patients who must make the final decision. What, they are asking, is the real story?

The "real" story is that the operation *does* relieve pain in 85 to 90 percent of the patients who have it. Even the surgery's severest critics admit that patients who were almost sedentary before revascularization are able to mow lawns, play tennis, jog and lead pain-free lives afterward. Their performance on stress tests documents improved exercise tolerance.

"The quality of life is important," says Deborah's Dr. Gerald Lemole. "Life is two-dimensional. It is not only how long you live, but how you live.

"If you ask a patient who has been incapacitated with

pain and is now free of it, he or she will tell you every time that this is the beginning of a new world, that it has opened new doors for him or her. You can't underestimate the importance of that. Nor can you ignore the economic drain created by persons who must see doctors all the time, hop in and out of hospitals and lose time from work."

Bernard P., fifty-eight, on whom Dr. Lemole operated several years ago, testifies that he "came through the operation perfectly. They were right when they told me I would have little trouble. I had almost no pain from the operation, and now I feel, not as good as before, but better than before. Before I couldn't do anything. I felt so tied down, and that is not my way of living. Now I feel free and happy, not afraid of activity and, best of all, without pain. I know there is a lot of controversy about the operation, but as far as I'm concerned, I'm happy I had it."

Genevieve T., who is sixty-two, is not so happy. "I didn't feel too bad while I was in the hospital after the surgery," she said. "But when I came home, I kept waiting to get my strength back. I expected to feel weak for a while, but I also expected that the weakness would go away.

"But I found that my energy was drained, and the incision in my chest hurt, and the incision in my leg hurt. After a few months, those pains got better, but the original angina came back. And it was even worse than before. I couldn't push a mop around my kitchen without getting the pain.

"In the beginning, my doctor thought I was complaining without cause. He thought I didn't have what he called 'a positive attitude.' But when they retested me a few months later, they saw that the grafts I had gotten had closed. So what good did it do me to have the surgery? No good. They advise that I have the operation again. But there is no way I'll do it. I'd rather live with the pain."

A recent report from the Cleveland Clinic described a survey of nearly 3,000 women who underwent coronary artery surgery. It found that the operative mortality was slightly higher and that graft patency and angina relief was less than in men. But the five- and ten-year longevity in both sexes was almost identical.

Many physicians agree that the attitude of the patient counts heavily, not only toward the success of the surgery, but in the decision to have the operation in the first place. "Pain," explains Dr. Lemole, "is a subjective thing. What is intolerable to one person is manageable to another."

Consider Fred P., fifty-four, Bernard's brother, who had a heart attack nineteen years ago when he was thirty-five and has had angina pains for the past six years.

"I get them often," he says. "If I walk a little too fast or eat a little too much or get excited . . . even during sex, I get them. Not a day goes by that I don't get the pains.

"About six or seven weeks ago, I had terrible pain that even my medication didn't relieve. The doctors put me in the hospital and wanted to do a test to see if I needed a bypass operation. I thought about it, but the next morning I felt fine. I checked myself out of the hospital.

"I've made up my mind that I'm not going to have the operation. I can still get around. I work every day. I'm not bedridden. I have some pain . . . I take some nitro [nitroglycerin, a medication often prescribed to relieve angina]. I'm satisfied.

"I don't want to go under the knife. The thought of getting cut up and down my legs and getting my chest opened up . . . it's not for me. Besides, I don't think it can cure what I've got."

Fred is correct. The heart-bypass surgery cannot cure his coronary artery disease. Cardiologists who treat patients with the condition and the surgeons who operate on them admit, if asked, that the disease is progressive. Surgery can bypass existing obstructions, but it cannot prevent additional ones from forming.

"I tell my patients that we are not taking away the disease, we are not curing the disease," says Dr. Horace MacVaugh of Philadelphia's Lankenau Hospital. Dr. MacVaugh and his surgical team perform more than 500 bypasses a year.

"I tell them that everyone is on a gradual downhill course, but that theirs is at a little sharper angle than that of the general population. With this operation, we take them off that curve and move them straight up and start them off again. From that point, they will probably go downhill again at about the same rate that they did before unless they can do something to alter their life-style, which may have contributed to the condition."

In that case, patients are wondering: Does it make sense to have the operation? Are the benefits worth the risks? Will it prolong my life?

3 WHICH TESTS MIGHT I NEED TO DIAGNOSE MY CONDITION?

Ruth B. is a seventy-two-year-old woman who has never experienced heart problems. She has a normal cholesterol level, low-to-normal blood pressure and has never smoked. However, she is complaining of chest pains that may be angina. And she has become short of breath at even the slightest exertion.

Walking quickly across her kitchen can bring on the breathlessness. So can climbing the stairs, eating a big meal or riding her bicycle three blocks to the shopping center. Her chest pains, however, are not typical of angina. For one thing, they are located over the heart, rather than beneath the breastbone, and they do not radiate to her shoulders, arms or neck. Sometimes, Ruth says, a moist heating pad will relieve her discomfort. Ruth's doctor ordered a *resting electrocardiogram* (the written record of a test that reveals important information about heart rhythm and condition of heart muscle), to be followed by a *nuclear study* (tests requiring injection of a dye, isotope, or similar substance) of her heart.

Peter L. is fifty-five, overweight, smokes two packs of cigarettes a day, has a blood pressure of 170/110 and has a cholesterol level of 410. He is experiencing symptoms which, according to his description, are typical angina.

His chest pain, which shoots to his arm and neck, comes
when he has exercised and is relieved when he rests. The
pains come three or four times a day and have compromised his ability to work and to enjoy life. Peter's cardiologist immediately ordered a *catheterization* of his heart.

Then there is Jonathan Z., who is forty-seven and has a
history remarkably similar to Peter's. He, too, weighs fifty
pounds too much, has been a heavy smoker but has just
given it up. He has high blood pressure, 180/120, which
has been difficult to control with medication. Jonathan has
an elevated cholesterol level—340—and his older brother
had a heart attack last year, from which he has recovered.
Jonathan's cardiologist said a heart catheterization may
be necessary. But first he hospitalized him and ordered a
stress test.

It is not surprising that patients are bewildered by the
dazzling array of studies that may be prescribed by their
doctors to diagnose their heart problems. They wonder
what they are, what they are supposed to show, how valuable they are and how risky they are. And they are curious
about why their brother-in-law who has angina has been
whisked to the catheterization laboratory, while their sister with the same condition has never had a test other
than a standard electrocardiogram.

The studies stir up as much controversy as does the
bypass operation itself. There are sharp and as yet irrecon-
cilable differences about the appropriateness of their use
on specific patients. And it is not uncommon for one doctor to order a test that another doctor will condemn as
having no value. There have even been accusations that
physicians will sometimes order their patients to have
studies that they don't need in order to justify the pur-
chase of expensive testing equipment. And there is a feeling that patients who go to a large teaching institution,
with a costly nuclear-medicine department, may find

themselves studied and tested a lot more than those who consult a physician unaffiliated with such a facility.

There is no question that the smorgasbord of testing instruments, with their ability to define precisely coronary artery disease, has revolutionized the practice of cardiology and contributed to a slowly decreasing rate of death from heart disease. But some of the tests have a degree of risk. Others look more ominous than they are because they involve a tangle of intricate space-age equipment that seems to be the stuff of which science fiction is made. Counters, scanners, monitors, ultrasound machines and computers proliferate.

Patients are entitled to understand the meaning of each test, what the doctor hopes to learn from it, and, most important, how it will influence the course of their treatment. Given this information, many patients will be able to ask their doctors the most pertinent questions, better understand the answers—perhaps, challenge them—and finally decide, in collaboration with their physicians, "Is this test necessary for me?"

Everyone agrees that for a person suffering with angina pain, no matter how mild, a thorough physical examination (which includes taking a detailed family history) is a critical first step, and one that can be done by a competent family physician. Dr. Vladir Maranhao, director of the adult cardiac-catheterization laboratories at Deborah Heart and Lung Center in New Jersey, estimates that a diagnosis can be made with 60 to 75 percent accuracy based on the history and physical examination alone. "I should have a suspicion of the diagnosis after a forty-five-minute examination," he says.

An examination of this kind will pick up, without expensive and intimidating testing, a number of risk factors that may determine the need for further testing. Weight, blood pressure, age, smoking history and questions about diet, exercise and family background are easily obtained and contribute heavily toward developing a suspected diagnosis.

Obviously, a man whose grandfather, father and brother have all had heart attacks would initiate more concern than a man with similar symptoms but a negative family history for heart attacks. But if the man without heart disease in his family was a heavy smoker, had alarmingly high blood pressure and was fifty-five, a vulnerable age, his risk would rise, and a physician would be more likely to investigate further.

Blood work, including the incriminating cholesterol and triglyceride levels, as well as measurements of high- and low-density lipoproteins and searches for a trace of sugar in the urine will reveal even more. An *electrocardiogram*, which can be administered in the GP's office (often by the physician's nurse), can pick up heart *arrhythmias* (irregularities in heartbeat) and spot damage from past heart attacks.

Damage from past heart attacks is significant for a person suffering from angina pain. "You know that one area of the heart is damaged by a previous heart attack," says Dr. Richard H. Helfant, professor of clinical medicine at the University of Pennsylvania Medical School and director of the mid-Atlantic Heart and Vascular Institute at Presbyterian University of Pennsylvania Medical Center. "So new angina tells you that the person has disease in at least one other vessel, which means that he has multivessel heart disease. If he suffers another heart attack, his mortality risk is increased because you are dealing with cumulative damage."

Together, this vital data can be translated into a "risk profile," a reasonable estimate of a patient's likelihood of having coronary artery disease.

However, what an individual physician does with this

information varies dramatically. Some physicians, such as Dr. J. Willis Hurst, chairman of the department of medicine at Emory University, says that he would send any patient with *new* angina symptoms for a heart catheterization and *angiogram* (the most aggressive of diagnostic and prognostic tests). "There is no other way that you can know for sure about the extent of the disease in the coronary arteries," says Dr. Hurst. He would not, however, have coronary arteriograms performed on all elderly patients.

Other physicians say that their decisions would be linked to a number of factors, including the person's age, sex, and degree of disability from the angina.

Dr. Robert Katz, for instance, a Philadelphia cardiologist, says, "If I were seeing a patient with typical *new* angina, and the patient were a man or woman over sixty-five and having mild symptoms, I would do a standard electrocardiogram [commonly known as an *ECG*]. If the ECG were normal and the patient had no discomfort at rest or after meals, I would advise him to lose weight if he were overweight, treat him for blood pressure if necessary and ask him to walk and swim, but not to lift heavy objects. I would not test him further at that time, but I would treat him medically and watch his symptoms."

If a patient with similar symptoms were younger, however, Dr. Katz would be more likely to perform, for starters, one of the noninvasive tests described below to determine how much exercise the patient could tolerate without getting chest pain or showing abnormalities on his electrocardiogram. The results of this test would determine whether further studies were needed.

Some physicians, although not all, would begin with an exercise *stress test*. This is an examination of the heart's ability to deliver blood containing oxygen to the heart muscles as they work harder and harder.

Exercise testing is big business in America, and many executives must take a stress test as a routine part of their mandated physical examination. It works this way: The patient rides on a stationary bicycle or runs in place on a treadmill while he or she is continually monitored for blood-pressure changes, pulse rate, the electrical activity of the heart and symptoms of heart or blood-vessel deficiencies.

The bicycle or treadmill begins slowly, then increases in speed every three minutes until it reaches a limit that is determined by the person's age. If symptoms—usually chest pains—appear before that time, the test is stopped. This reaction would be defined as positive.

Physicians are looking particularly at the level of a specific part of the electrocardiogram called the ST segment. Certain fluctuations in this segment can signify the shortage of oxygen to the heart muscle and arouse suspicion that there are clogged arteries.

Normal response to a stress test will be elevated blood pressure (to a certain point) during exercise, no chest pain and no depression in that strategic ST segment of the electrocardiogram. A decrease in blood pressure, pain early in the test (which often indicates that the vital left ventricle of the heart is not functioning properly), depression of the ST segment greater than two millimeters or the development of a persistent arrhythmia of the ventricle could be dangerous signs that may indicate the need for further investigation.

A significant ST segment depression early in the electrocardiogram could lead to the suspicion that the patient has disease of his left main coronary artery (which is critical), the left anterior descending artery or disease in more than one vessel of his heart.

The problem with the stress test, however, and the reason that many doctors have little faith in it is its poor reliability. Only 70 percent of patients who have coronary artery disease will have a positive stress test, and, conversely, 30 percent of people with the disease will have a negative stress test.

If that were not perplexing enough, 10 percent of people who do not have coronary artery disease will have positive stress tests. And if the person is a woman, especially a younger woman, the number of false positive tests increases.

For example, of 1,000 fifty-five-year-old men, all with a 10 percent risk of having coronary artery disease, 100 are likely to actually have the condition. Of the 100, only 70 will have a positive stress test. Thirty of those who have the condition will not demonstrate it on a stress test. And ninety men who do not have the condition will have stress-test results indicating that they do have it.

This means that, of the original 1,000 men, there will probably be 160 positive stress tests, 70 from men who have coronary artery disease and 90 from men who do not.

Dr. James Forrester and his colleague, Dr. George Diamond, who have created a stress laboratory in Los Angeles which computerizes risk factors and stress-test results, emphasize that the test can only measure probabilities but cannot be definite about pinpointing coronary artery disease in an individual. "In our original group of one thousand fifty-five-year-old men, each of the one hundred sixty who had a positive stress test has a predicted statistical likelihood of forty-four percent of having coronary artery disease," says Dr. Forrester. "And that doesn't tell you much."

What Dr. Forrester does is try to make the results reveal more. He plots the pretest risk (based on the risk factors uncovered in physical examinations and laboratory tests) together with the post-test risk evidenced by the stress test. This gives him a more reliable measure of the individual's probability of having coronary artery disease.

Consider, for instance, a man with a 50 percent chance of having coronary artery disease before he takes a stress test. His test is positive. This raises his likelihood of having the disease to 86 percent. If his test is negative, it lowers his risk to 22 percent. These results may help a physician and his patient determine how much additional testing, if any, ought to be done.

In addition to its questionable accuracy, the stress test cannot be used in patients who suffer from shortness of breath. These patients would become breathless before the stress were increased enough to show changes in the electrocardiogram.

And in patients who have already shown abnormalities in a resting electrocardiogram, many physicians feel that an exercise test is of no additional value. They say that in such cases, the patient is beginning the exercise test with irregularities already recorded. This eliminates the opportunity to see at what point in the exercise the problem begins. And this information is significant.

The risk of taking a stress test is small. A study of 170,000 tests revealed that for every 10,000 persons tested, one may die and two or three may require hospitalization. Occasionally, emergency treatment is needed.

Drs. Jaime Benrey, Wayne E. Dear and Denton A. Cooley of the Texas Heart Institute, St. Luke's Episcopal and Texas Children's Hospitals in Houston describe a fifty-four-year-old man who did require emergency treatment after suffering a heart attack subsequent to a stress test.

The patient—we'll call him Michael—was admitted to the Texas Heart Institute after experiencing chest pain, which he described as a burning sensation sometimes related to physical activity, but which did not radiate to his arm or neck. He was a moderately heavy cigarette smoker but had no other pertinent risk factors. His blood pressure was 130/76, his heart rate was a normal 72 beats per minute and his resting electrocardiogram was normal. *Arteriography* (an invasive test which shows blocked arteries) of his heart showed that he had a blockage in his left anterior descending coronary artery and in his right coronary artery.

Michael's physicians wanted to check his performance on exercise and ordered a treadmill test, which increased in intensity every few minutes. Surprisingly, considering that his angiogram (a procedure that tests for coronary artery disease) had already shown significant blockages in two arteries, Michael experienced no chest pain during his exercise, nor did his electrocardiogram show any changes, either during the test or for ten minutes after the test was completed. But fourteen minutes after the exercise, Michael had a heart attack and was admitted within two hours as an emergency case for bypass surgery. The results of his operation were good.

While exercise testing is usually a benign procedure, the doctors point out that "no test procedure is absolutely and invariably safe." That's why it is critical that the test be administered by a specialist who is professionally competent and who carefully monitors and watches the patient throughout the procedure.

Among more than 7,000 people who had such stress tests at the Texas Heart Institute, Michael is the only person who experienced a heart attack during or shortly after his exercise testing. And most studies suggest that the risk of death or heart attack is extremely low—from 0.1 percent to 0.4 percent. So it is rarely the risk that keeps doctors from ordering the tests . . . it is more likely to be the vague—some say useless—results that influence their decisions.

Dr. Forrester argues, however, that "the assessment of pretest risk is going to be increasingly important as we enter the era of cost-effective decisions. We will have to use multiple tests, beginning with low cost, simple assessment of risk and progressing to more costly tests in a patient without symptoms, only when the risk is high," he says.

Consider a forty-eight-year-old man with atypical angina pains (pains that correlate somewhat, but not precisely, to chest pain caused by blocked arteries), a systolic blood pressure of 150, a cholesterol level of 350, a non-smoker, nondiabetic and with a normal resting electrocardiogram. Dr. Forrester's computers give this man a 62 percent pretest risk of having coronary artery disease. But his ECG during exercise, a test of intermediate cost, shows ST segment depression of two millimeters, which is a significant finding. With this new information, the computer reveals that his probability of having atherosclerosis has risen to 97.2 percent.

Should he have further, more expensive diagnostic testing—a nuclear study, for instance? No, says Dr. Forrester. With this high a probability of having disease, the man will most likely be recommended for a catheterization of his heart so that the location and extent of his blockages can be seen. A catheterization is a test to determine, among other things, the location and extent of blockages in the coronary arteries.

Another man, fifty-five, has atypical chest pain, a cholesterol level of 250, blood pressure of 140, is not diabetic, does not smoke and has an abnormal resting electrocardiogram. His pretest risk is 14 percent, according to the computer. His stress test is positive, showing one millimeter ST segment depression. After the test, the computer raises the odds to 40 percent.

Does this man need additional nuclear tests? "Absolutely," says Dr. Forrester. He has a 40 percent likelihood of having atherosclerosis. There is not much confidence in his stress-test results because his resting electrocardiogram was abnormal, thus reducing the validity of his exercise-test result. Another noninvasive study might be considered, since the result would give the patient a very low or very high probability of disease. Or, depending on the doctor, the patient could skip the in-between steps and proceed to have his heart catheterized.

It is a decision usually made by the physician, based on his interpretation of the data and his or her own inclinations toward aggressive testing. In the case described above, the opinions of doctors would differ sharply. Dr. Forrester feels it is seldom justified to refer a person to catheterization, the most expensive test, unless there is a ninety percent or greater chance of coronary artery disease.

"How you decide whether to go on to further testing is important," says Dr. Forrester. "It reminds me," he quips, "of a cartoon I once saw. Two weather forecasters were talking, and one said to the other: 'There is a forty percent chance of rain tonight. And there is a ten percent chance I know what I'm talking about.'

"It isn't just your estimate of the patient's disease probability as shown by the computer," says Dr. Forrester, "but the confidence you have in that estimate."

The next step, if results of a stress test indicate it is necessary, might be a *thallium scan.* This is a nuclear test, sometimes administered in conjunction with a stress test, during which the patient exercises on a treadmill or bicycle just as he would for a stress test. All the time he is exercising, he is monitored by a continuous electrocardiogram, and his pulse, blood pressure and heart rate are being recorded. But at the peak of exercise, the patient is injected in the arm with thallium 20, a radioisotope. As the thallium circulates through the blood, through the coronary arteries to the heart muscle, a specially equipped gamma scintillation camera, which has been placed over his chest, scans the progress of the thallium. These signals are translated by a computer into a picture of the way the thallium is distributed in the heart muscle. Where thallium does not circulate or has poor circulation to the muscle, a "cold spot" will appear in the picture, indicating that the coronary artery supplying blood to that area is blocked.

Unlike the stress test, false positives are infrequent, and thallium scans are extremely sensitive. If there is coronary artery disease present, the thallium scan will almost always pick it up.

"The thallium scan is highly reliable," says Dr. Katz. "From it, you can deduce which arteries are involved. For instance, when the chest pains begin at a particular point in the exercise and the ECG records changes in the heart's anterior wall, you would strongly suspect that there was a blockage in the left main artery of the heart or in the left anterior descending artery. If that occurred, I would be more likely to move the patient on to a heart catheterization."

However, the thallium scan, like the stress test, cannot be administered to the patient who is short of breath because the stress would force cessation of the test before significant changes could occur.

Another study, useful to measure the flow of blood to a given area of the left ventricle (the chamber of the heart which pumps blood to all parts of the body, including the heart itself) is called a *nuclear ventriculogram.* Here, another radioactive isotope, technitium, is injected into the arm. The patient lies on a table beneath a camera which scans his chest and creates, via a computer, a picture of the wall motion of the left ventricle. If the technitium does not move as well through one segment of the ventricle as the others, this may indicate that the arteries supplying that segment are narrowed and not providing enough oxygen.

The test reveals what, in the medical world, is known as the "ejection fraction" of the heart. This means that during the resting period of the heart's pumping process (the diastole), a certain amount of blood goes into the ventricle. During the pumping period (systole), it is squeezed out or "ejected." A normal "ejection fraction" is about 50 percent, indicating that the heart muscle is pumping efficiently. An ejection fraction of 70 to 80 percent is excellent, and, of course, an ejection fraction of 10 or 20 percent would be considered dangerous. It would indicate that the contractual ability of the heart is very poor.

This information is important for patients considering bypass surgery. Some physicians will not operate on anyone with a poor ejection fraction. They consider it too risky. Other physicians, however, such as Dr. Dudley Johnson of Wisconsin, have performed surgery on many such patients with excellent results.

Like the thallium scan, the nuclear ventriculogram is 90 to 94 percent accurate. Neither test has side effects. The radiation dose is just slightly more than that delivered by a chest X ray, and there is no pain involved in taking the tests. Disadvantages have to do mainly with the high cost because of expensive equipment and the need for skilled personnel to administer the tests.

The bottom line in testing is the *coronary catheterization* and *coronary angiogram*. Persons who are not being tested for the presence of coronary artery disease may undergo catheterization without the angiographic studies. This means that the pressure from the chambers of the heart will be measured, blood samples from the chambers of the heart will be taken and dye will be injected into the left and/or right ventricles to check the "ejection fraction." This kind of testing is done on patients with congenital heart disease, rheumatic diseases of the heart or valve problems.

But when someone is suspected of having coronary artery disease, the coronary angiogram (also called an arteriogram) is performed at the same time, and it is this procedure many patients say they most fear. But Emory's Dr. Willis Hurst calls the coronary arteriogram "the greatest advance of the century in heart diagnostic technology."

The coronary arteriogram is a method of visualizing the coronary arteries and pinpointing the locations and extent of blockages. It was developed in the late 1950s by Dr. F. Mason Sones, Jr., of the Cleveland Clinic. It happened by accident. Dr. Sones was catheterizing a patient's left ventricle, but the catheter slipped into the right coronary artery, and the right coronary arteries showed up on his screen. Subsequently, Dr. Sones developed another catheter that was more easily able to wend its way into the coronary opening, refined his methods and created the diagnostic procedure which has changed the course of treatment for heart patients.

The procedure works this way: a catheter is inserted into an artery in the arm or the groin (many doctors prefer the groin because it is more comfortable for the patient) and snakes its way up into the heart. The catheter is guided into position with the help of a large television monitor (hooked up to X-ray equipment placed above and below the table on which the patient is lying) on which an image of the heart is projected. Dye is then injected directly into the patient's coronary arteries (through the catheter), and the flow of the dye, projected onto the television screen, shows the location, pattern and extent of the blockages. This procedure is critical in determining the prognosis of the patient, and it is one that must be done before anyone can undergo heart-bypass surgery. It becomes the surgeon's road map in the operating room.

Approximately one-third of the patients catheterized end up having surgery. The others either do not have coronary artery disease or have disease too extensive or not extensive enough for surgery.

The coronary arteriogram is not, however, without risk. There is a slight chance that cardiac arrest may occur during the procedure, and in rare cases, a stroke and/or heart attack may occur. Other risks include allergic reaction to the dye, local trauma to the blood vessels, local infections and occasionally the loss of a peripheral pulse.

However, in skilled hands, the risk is minimal, from almost 0 to 0.18 percent. "Many patients fear the catheterization, but in the right hands, there is practically no risk," says Deborah Hospital's Dr. Maranhao. Dr. Maranhao's hands have performed more than 25,000 catheterizations in twenty-three years, and his fatality rate is 0.18 percent.

Although there have been instances when the catheterization has been performed on an out-patient basis, most physicians require a brief hospital stay, from one to five days. Before the test is performed, other studies, such as electrocardiogram, blood work, chest X rays and, when indicated, some noninvasive heart studies (such as *echocardiogram* which shows the structural functioning of the heart by transmitting ultrasound into the body and recording the echoes returning from the heart's surface), and nuclear scans during rest and exercise, may be ordered.

The catheterization lasts from approximately twenty minutes to one and a half hours, depending on the severity of the case. During that time the patient lies on the padded X-ray table. He or she will be awake throughout to cooperate with the medical team regarding breathing and coughing. Local anesthesia is used to avoid pain at the puncture or incision sites (where the catheter is inserted). The dye used to visualize the heart and its vessels produces a warm, sometimes uncomfortable sensation, which disappears within a few seconds.

After the catheterization, the patient is sometimes asked to remain in bed for twenty-four hours. He may shower, eat regular food and will usually feel little or no discomfort. If an incision was performed, stitches are removed a few days later. If there is an area of hardening in the area of the incision, warm compresses are applied several times a day for a few days.

Is the procedure more dangerous if it is performed on an out-patient? Dr. Earl S. Perrigo, a cardiologist from Toledo, Ohio, says no. He is one of three authors of a paper called "Twenty Month Experience in Outpatient Cardiac Catheterization," which describes 224 consecutive cardiac catheterizations with coronary angiography which were performed at the Michienzi Medical Center in Sandusky, Ohio, in 1974. The center is a nonhospital, out-patient medical clinic which performed 1,300 cardiac catheterizations between 1974 and 1980.

Of the 224 out-patients, there were 1.8 percent major complications (weak radial pulse, ventricular fibrillation), 6.3 percent minor complications (transient minor arrhythmias, minor allergic reaction to dye) and no deaths. These results are similar to those reported in four published university studies of inpatient cardiac catheterization.

Many patients preferred the out-patient procedure because they did not have to spend too much time away from their families and felt less anxiety when not hospitalized.

Some physicians, such as Dr. Stephen E. Epstein, Chief

of Cardiology at the National Heart, Lung and Blood Institute of the National Institutes of Health, do not believe that the arteriogram is necessary in most instances to diagnose the existence of coronary artery disease. He says that the noninvasive tests (described earlier in this chapter) and the history and symptoms of the patient are usually enough to establish a diagnosis of coronary artery disease. He cites an illustration: A patient with atypical chest pain, with some but not all of the features of classical angina, has about a 50 percent pretest likelihood of having clogged arteries. A positive stress test in this patient still provides equivocal results. So does a negative stress test. But a nuclear study, which is highly reliable, can usually rule in or out the diagnosis of coronary artery disease.

"In such circumstances," says Dr. Epstein, "the results of a second noninvasive study, added to the results of the first study, if concordant, establish the presence or absence of disease with a high degree of certainty. Hence, with current noninvasive testing, it is usually unnecessary to consider using coronary angiography to establish whether or not coronary artery disease exists."

However, the results of the catheterization can be crucial because they reveal information that cannot be gleaned from any other tests currently in use. "Once a patient has described his symptoms and they are clearly classic effort angina (chest pain on exertion) there is no noninvasive diagnostic test which will substantially increase your diagnostic accuracy," says University of Pennsylvania's Dr. Richard Helfant.

And all doctors agree that there is often a poor correlation between the symptoms of coronary artery disease and the extent of the condition. Some patients go from heart attack to heart attack without ever experiencing angina. They probably have blockages but, for some reason, do not feel any pain or they experience pain of which they are tolerant. And half or more of male deaths because of coronary artery disease appears in angina-free patients.

In addition, patients with mild angina may have strategically located, life-threatening blockages, and some with severe discomfort may have cleaner arteries that are not at the time life-threatening. "Patients die because of obstructions in their arteries, not because of angina," says Milwaukee's Dr. Dudley Johnson. "That's why a study of the coronary anatomy is critical."

The principal reason, many physicians agree, for a coronary angiogram is to determine a patient's prognosis and to decide whether he or she is a candidate for a bypass operation.

So again, a patient with *new, classic angina* (which most doctors call *"unstable" angina*) could receive medical treatment and remain under careful scrutiny by his physician; he could receive a series of tests that might or might not land him on the catheterization table. Or he could go directly from his physician's office to the hospital or laboratory for an invasive study of his coronary arteries.

But some physicians, among them University of Alabama's Dr. Thomas James, a former president of the American Heart Association, do not like to refer to new angina as "unstable" and are reluctant to proceed with costly testing procedures. "How do you know that new angina, if treated medically, will not become stable?" he asks. Stable angina is the term used to describe angina of six months' or longer duration that has not increased in intensity or interfered with a person's life-style. "You don't give it a chance," he says. "And statistics show that thirty-five percent of patients with angina quit having it eventually anyway."

When a patient experiences symptoms that are not classic angina or has had angina for more than six months with no change, the approach by doctors is dramatically different than that for those with new angina.

"There is a difference between people who have had angina pectoris for six months, a year, two years, five years, which has not changed at all and who are able to perform all of their activities, and those with new symptoms [unstable angina]," says Emory's Dr. Willis Hurst. "The longer a person has had the condition and the longer it has remained unchanged, the less likely you would be to do aggressive testing," he says.

If the pain is atypical angina, meaning that it is not located where angina pains usually are, or that it does not move to the arms or shoulders, or that it does not appear with activity and vanish with rest, the procedure would depend on several factors. The age and sex of the patient would count heavily.

"If I had a patient with atypical chest pain and the patient were a male between the ages of thirty and fifty-five [a vulnerable age group], I would be more suspicious than I would if it were a woman," says Dr. Robert Katz of Philadelphia. "I would be more likely to proceed to a thallium study and on to catheterization if those findings warranted it. The more atypical the pain is, the less likely I am to do anything, but with a male, if I have any suspicion at all, I would be inclined to move on to, at the least, nuclear tests."

In premenopausal females, atypical chest pain often tends to be unrelated to the heart, so doctors will search for other reasons. The pain could be caused by *esophagitis* (inflammation of the esophagus), a problem with the cervical spine, the gall bladder or *costochondritis* (an inflammation of the rib cage). "If the pain were bothersome enough, I might do an exercise thallium test," Dr. Katz says.

In women who are postmenopausal, even atypical chest pain would be looked on with greater concern and would generally be treated the same as for men with similar complaints. The tests prescribed would depend on how convinced the doctor was that the pain was actually related to the heart.

Patients with unstable angina—not because it is new, but because it has grown in intensity and frequency, or is intense and prolonged while at rest with little or no response to medication, or is experienced within thirty days after a heart attack—present a dilemma for doctors. Most would order a series of tests, with the possibility of a catheterization lurking in the background. The results of the earlier tests would help determine whether angiography was required.

What about the patient who has had a heart attack but feels well afterward, with no pain? Should a catheterization be performed automatically? Wisconsin's Dr. Dudley Johnson says yes.

"We think it is important to do a catheterization after an infarction to see what is really happening in those arteries. For someone who is, maybe, eighty years old or has a medical reasons why it would be unwise, we might not do it. But otherwise, we would strongly recommend it."

"No," says Dr. Katz. "At our present state of knowledge, if a patient feels well after the heart attack and there is no suspicion of left main coronary disease, I do not see the sense of studies after infarction, unless there should be further pain. There may, of course, be exceptions. If, for instance, a patient has four brothers with heart attacks who died at forty-two, the catheterization might be used as a diagnostic test."

"Maybe," says NIH's Dr. Stephen Epstein. "During the first year following an acute myocardial infarction [heart attack], ten to fifteen percent of patients will die. Several studies have identified subgroups that are at high or low risk of sudden death. Hence, we have to wonder whether identification of high-risk patients, after heart attack, can lead to more effective therapeutic approaches."

Unfortunately, definitive data are not yet available. But it is known that most patients who die in the twelve months following a heart attack seem to have impaired function of their left ventricle; this has been documented by nuclear studies. Their "ejection fraction" when they are discharged from the hospital is less than 40 percent (normal is 50 percent), and studies obtained shortly after the onset of their heart-attack symptoms also demonstrate defects of more than 40 percent in the left ventricle. In addition, patients who show an ST segment depression of two millimeters or more on exercise testing prior to discharge from the hospital also have a high one-year mortality rate. The statistics look like this:

- Heart-attack patients who have ejection fractions of less than 40 percent when released from the hospital have a 20 percent mortality rate within a year.
- Persons with defects of the left ventricle in excess of 40 percent shortly after heart-attack symptoms appear (as demonstrated by thallium imaging studies) have a first-year mortality rate of 85 percent.
- Patients exhibiting an ST segment depression of more than two millimeters on a predischarge exercise test have a 20 percent mortality in the first year.

The effects of surgery on the prognosis of patients in these high-risk groups are not known; however, Dr. Epstein believes that the high one-year mortality justifies coronary angiography in those patients in order to consider the possibility of surgery.

"I wouldn't recommend that everybody in the United

States who has a heart attack be angiogramed," says Dr. Floyd Loop of the Cleveland Clinic. "It would depend on the age, seriousness of the heart attack, whether chest pain or other symptoms occur after the heart attack. But for a person who is feeling well, it is a decision based on the judgment of the attending cardiologist."

Because so many patients who experience heart attacks have had no warnings in the form of angina, some physicians, such as Dr. Dudley Johnson, believe that a stress test should be performed from time to time on persons who are older than forty. However, other doctors do not agree.

"The stress test is not a good screening tool for normal people, but we have nothing else better right now," says University of Pennsylvania's Dr. Richard Helfant. "The trap you get into is that we can see a positive test in a patient without symptoms and send him for an angiogram, as a result. If it is positive, he winds up on the operating table. So you have a patient who has been catheterized, bypassed and may be worse off than he was before."

Other diagnostic tests are being pursued, and many physicians are hopeful that within the next decade or two, noninvasive methods of visualizing the coronary arteries may be developed. Meanwhile, a number of techniques are helping to more specifically diagnose heart problems.

One is Position Emission Tomography (PET) which permits a multidimensional look into the body. It has been used to better understand the metabolism and blood flow in the brain, but a team at the Washington University School of Medicine in St. Louis has aimed it toward the heart. While PET cannot peer directly into the coronary arteries, it can evaluate the health of the surrounding tissue to which the artery supplies blood.

If the tissue around a blocked artery is healthy, indicating that collaterals have built up to compensate for the artery blockage, it may be possible to avoid an operation.

PET is unique in that it can identify an area of heart muscle that is starving and is about to die.

A new scanner at the Mayo Clinic—called "dynamic spatial reconstructor"—can take three-dimensional images of the heart the size of a basketball, up to 15,000 pictures a second as it circles the body. It is purely a research tool which may be available for patient use in the future. Its main purpose will be to define heart, lung and circulatory function.

And a new method of photographing the heart called "digital subtraction angiography" is under study at the Cleveland Clinic. The procedure, which was developed by physicists working independently at the Universities of Arizona and Wisconsin, is considered an important advance in the visualization of the cardiovascular system. Through this method, a simple intravenous injection in the arm and fifteen minutes of the patient's time are all that are required. There is no X-ray film used, just a link between a digital computer, a fluoroscope and X-ray machines. The equipment sees through bony and soft tissue, while providing a computerized picture of what is happening in the arteries. Although the technique is being used to study wall motion of the heart and to identify congenital heart disease, it is not yet available to visualize the coronary arteries.

Other laboratories are working with a digital computer system that is able to estimate the dimensions of the clogged portion of a coronary artery. The computer calculates the resistance to blood flow that the blockage is causing and estimates the severity of narrowing. The technique, called "quantitative coronary arteriography," was developed by Dr. Bruce Gregory Brown, associate professor of medicine at the University of Washington at Seattle in collaboration with Dr. Harold T. Dodge. Dr. Brown says, "We take the information from coronary arteriograms and quantify it in a way that makes it much more precise." This information can be used to determine which factors in a patient's arteriogram are predictive of the effectiveness of bypass surgery.

The technique has also been used to demonstrate the progression of a specific blockage. For instance, Dr. Brown has followed 600 blockages in forty-seven patients. When he repeated their arteriograms after eighteen months, he found that approximately 15 percent of the blockages progressed and about 5 percent regressed. But when he separated the patients into two groups—one with high cholesterol and one with normal cholesterol, he learned that those with high cholesterol experienced a greater likelihood of disease progression. "This clearly shows that in people who have high cholesterol levels, coronary artery lesions are more likely to get worse and less likely to improve," Dr. Brown says.

He found also that the more severe the blockages were, the more likely they were to get worse.

As promising as this technique is, it is still too expensive and too time-consuming to be used on a widespread basis. And a reliable substitute for heart catheterization and angiography is probably not going to be available for at least ten years.

Meanwhile, fewer patients are content to do what they once did—place their confidence and their bodies in the hands of a physician and follow his or her advice without a whimper or a question. They look for second and third opinions. And a steadily growing group of savvy patients insists on understanding the reasons for doctors' decisions and even suggests alternatives that may be more palatable.

When deliberating about a specific test that a physician

has recommended, these are the key factors a patient should remember:

- Physicians will make testing recommendations based on their experience, attitudes and knowledge of the field. They will reflect their own inclinations—aggressive or conservative—toward the practice of cardiac medicine.
- Where the patient's problem is clear-cut and unequivocal, there will be a lot of agreement among doctors. Where it is not, there can be many approaches, and there is as yet no certain evidence that any one is superior.
- The pain associated with coronary artery disease (angina) does not always correlate with the extent of the condition. Someone with mild pain, or even no pain, could have extensive disease affecting strategic arteries, and, conversely, a person with severe pain may not have disease that is widespread and life-threatening.
- While statistics are important in describing the probability of coronary artery disease in a given population, they may not be accurate in pinpointing the condition in a specific patient. For instance, while it is true that a thirty-year-old woman with atypical chest pain probably does not have angina, a particular thirty-year-old woman with that symptom could defy the statistics and have angina that demands attention.
- The more risk factors a person has, the more likely a physician will be to suggest aggressive tests.
- A coronary angiogram can indeed be risky, but the risk is small when it is performed by a skilled physician with a lot of experience.
- While many tests can rule in or out the probability of coronary artery disease, the angiogram is the *only* test that can identify precisely which arteries are blocked,

how serious the blockages are and how many arteries are affected. It is a test that *must* be done if heart-bypass surgery is under consideration.

Questions to which patients should have answers and which will contribute to their decisions about testing are:

What are my symptoms like?
· Are they classic angina?
· How long have I had them?
· Are they growing worse?
· Perhaps most important, are they keeping me from living the kind of life I prefer?

What are my risk factors?
· Do I have high blood pressure?
· How high is it?
· Have I taken, and am I still taking, medication to control it?
· Am I diabetic?
· Am I or have I ever been a smoker?
· How much do I smoke?
· What is my cholesterol level?
· If it is high, how high?
· What is my triglyceride level?
· Do I watch my diet, limiting my intake of fats and sugars?
· *And finally, what contribution toward better knowledge of my condition will each test—whether stress test, thallium test, ventriculogram, angiogram— afford? How will the results alter the course of treatment for me?*

Patients should ask for the following information after each test they take:

Resting Electrocardiogram
· Was the test normal?
· Is there evidence of a past heart attack?

- If so, how extensive is the area of damage?
- Are there ST segment depressions? How severe are they? (Depressions of two millimeters or more can be worrisome.)
- Are there arrythmias?
- What did the electrocardiogram reveal that indicates further testing is needed?

Stress Test
- At what point in the stress test (after how many minutes of exercise) did my chest pains begin?
- At what point in the stress test (after how many minutes of exercise) were there changes in the electrocardiogram?
- Did my blood pressure rise appropriately during the exercise? Or did it drop?
- Based on my risk factors, symptoms and results of the stress test, what is the probability that I have coronary artery disease?

Thallium Scan
- Were there "cold spots" on the picture of the heart muscle?
- Which arteries may be blocked, based on the results of this test?
- Is there any suspicion of how much blockage may be present?

Nuclear Ventriculogram
- What is the "ejection fraction" of my heart? Remember, 50 percent is normal. Anything below that may be significant in terms of the function of the heart muscle.

Catheterization and Angiogram
- Do I have clogged arteries?
- Which arteries are clogged?
- What is the percentage of blockage in each artery? (Lesions that are less than 50 percent are not considered to require surgery.)
- Do I have left main disease?

- Do I have a significant blockage of the left anterior descending artery close to the beginning of the artery?
- What do my distal vessels (vessels beyond the area of blockage) look like? Are they clogged? If so, are they operable?
- What is my ventricular function (my "ejection fraction")?

When all of the questions have been answered and all of the information is collected, the biggest riddle of all is: What do I do with what I know? How do I weigh the opinions of physicians who may differ? How indeed do I help decide (considering the opinion of my physician) whether I am a candidate for heart-bypass surgery?

4 AM I A CANDIDATE FOR BYPASS SURGERY?

Stella M., a fifty-two-year-old accountant who lives near Milwaukee, is confused. She has just had a series of tests, including a coronary catheterization and angiogram. She has talked with three doctors and received three different opinions about what she should do.

It started a few weeks ago when Stella, who is married and has three children—two sons and a daughter—began to experience an uncomfortable, clutching sensation in her chest. Gradually, her pain became more intense and occurred more frequently. Sometimes she felt as though she were strangling.

Her family physician sent her to a prominent cardiologist who first took her history. He learned that Stella has high blood pressure, for which she takes medication. Even so, her pressure sometimes soars to 180/105. She is diabetic and about forty pounds overweight. She has never smoked, and her cholesterol level is 300, a little high. Her father had a heart attack when he was sixty-two but recovered and is still living, with no symptoms of heart disease. Stella's electrocardiogram is normal.

The cardiologist then ordered a thallium stress test. When Stella had been exercising on the treadmill for a few minutes, changes began to appear on her electrocardiogram, and she had moderate chest discomfort. There were two "cold spots," indicating poor circulation to the heart muscle.

She was then sent to the nuclear-medicine department of the hospital for a ventriculogram. This test revealed that Stella had a good "ejection fraction," 60 percent, which meant that her left ventricle was functioning effectively.

Based on the results of the thallium test, Stella's family history, risk factors (high blood pressure, diabetes and overweight) and, most important, her symptoms, her physician urged her to have a catheterization and an angiogram. Results showed that she had an 80 percent blockage in her right coronary artery, a 90 percent blockage in her circumflex artery and a 40 percent blockage in her left anterior descending artery.

(Blood is sent to the heart muscle by the left and right coronary arteries. The left coronary artery divides shortly after its origin into the left anterior descending artery and the circumflex artery. The left anterior descending supplies a large part of the heart wall between the two ventricles and a large portion of the front wall of the left ventricle. The circumflex artery supplies the back of the left ventricle, and the right coronary artery transmits blood to the right ventricle and to parts of the back of the left ventricle.)

Since blockages of 40 percent are not significant enough to convince most doctors that surgery is warranted, Stella was said to have "two-vessel" disease.

Her cardiologist strongly recommended surgery, telling her that her condition was life-threatening and that her left anterior descending artery, now 40 percent blocked, was certain to deteriorate. He felt she was a good candidate for surgery because her "ejection fraction" was satisfactory, although her diabetes, extra weight, and the fact that she was a woman increased her surgical risk a little.

Stella consulted a surgeon who said he would do three bypasses. He would not normally perform surgery just to bypass a 40 percent blockage, but while he was "in there," he would graft that one too, because he felt that the more complete the revascularization, the better the outlook for Stella.

But Stella was not satisfied with one cardiologist's opinion. She had heard about the controversy over the bypass operation, and besides, she was fearful of undergoing so serious a procedure. "I shudder when I think about it," she says. "All of those tubes, and spending hours in an operating room under anesthesia. It scares me. Besides, my symptoms seemed to be under control with the medicine the cardiologist gave me." Since Stella was not in great pain, she waited two weeks for an appointment with another doctor to get a second opinion.

The new cardiologist was not as eager to rush Stella into surgery. He felt that two-vessel disease could often be controlled with drugs, and he was not certain that Stella would add years to her life if she underwent an operation. He wanted to try first to achieve better control over her blood pressure, lower her cholesterol and encourage her to lose weight. "If you do those things, the course of your angina may change," he told her. He recommended that Stella be placed on a medical regimen and be watched closely. If, however, her symptoms worsened and interfered with her way of life, she would require reappraisal.

Stella was willing, but her husband was skeptical. Several of his friends had had bypass surgery and felt marvelous. They were back on the golf course, full of energy, and their operations were only a dim memory. He wanted his wife to see his best friend's surgeon.

This doctor had still another recommendation. He felt

that Stella should have the operation, but he would do only two bypasses. "The 40 percent lesion in your left anterior descending artery does not require surgery," he told her. "I don't believe in doing more bypasses than you need. Let's do a double-vessel bypass."

By this time, understandably, Stella was confused, anxious and frustrated. How could three competent and respected physicians, given the same information about the same patient, differ so dramatically in their recommendations for treatment? And how could she possibly know which was the correct decision?

Stella's dilemma is not unusual. More patients each year are finding that physicians can have sharply different opinions about how their cases should be handled. One schedules a patient for surgery. Another sends him home with a bottle of little white pills.

"It's true," agrees Wisconsin's Dr. Dudley Johnson. "If a patient is not happy with what he hears from one doctor, he can always find another who will tell him something else."

That is why more patients, perplexed, distressed and frightened, seek to unravel the mystique that surrounds the bypass operation. They insist on a clearer understanding of just who are the "best" candidates for surgery. They want to know when it is indeed critical to agree without delay to an operation, and when it may be more judicious to bide their time. They need to know which questions to ask and how to interpret the answers. And because the controversy over the bypass operation is still so heated, they grope for clear explanations, so that they can become competent participants in their own health care.

The problem is that there is no perfect way to compare the long-term effects of bypass surgery with medical treatment. Each method that has been attempted has had its failures.

For instance, *retrospective matched studies* review previously observed patients. This method can compare the effect of surgery in the past ten years with the effect of medical management in the previous decade. However, there are problems:

1. Surgical techniques have improved dramatically since 1970, so that results and mortality figures from early in the decade would be quite different from those applicable later in the decade.
2. Medical management has improved also, and in recent years, physicians have become more effective in treating patients medically.
3. Consideration needs to be given to the kind of medical management each patient received and whether the patient adhered to it.
4. While the two groups of patients may have similar coronary anatomies, they may not be identical in terms of other characteristics (to be discussed later in this chapter) that affect survival.

Prospective matched studies enter patients into either a medical-treatment plan or a surgical plan as they are observed. Problems here are:

1. There may be bias in assigning a patient to either plan. For example, a more seriously ill person could be assigned to surgery, while a mildly ill individual, who could be expected to do well, could be assigned to medical care.
2. The same medical management is not used in all patients; that which is appropriate for one patient may not be suitable for another. And doctors vary in the medical treatment they prescribe.

3. Critical characteristics of patients other than coro-
    nary anatomies are not always considered.

The prospective randomized study, which seems to be
the best method, has its drawbacks too. It is conducted by
randomly assigning patients, during a given time period,
to either medical care or surgery. This method eliminates
any bias in patient selection. However, there are other
problems.

1. As is true in other studies, surgical techniques and
    medical care have both progressed, and the studies
    may not accurately reflect results being achieved cur-
    rently.
2. Some patients who are randomized to medical care
    will have to cross over to surgery because they do not
    respond.
3. If several medical centers participate in such a study,
    there is no certainty that the surgical teams in each
    center will be equally skilled. In heart surgery, the
    skill of the surgical team correlates closely to opera-
    tive and late (more than thirty days after surgery)
    mortality.

The tendency has been that studies coming out of centers that do significant numbers of bypass operations, such
as the Cleveland Clinic and the Texas Heart Institute in
Houston, reflect the efficacy of surgery to relieve pain and
prolong life. Other studies, such as those done by the
European Collaborative Group, the Veterans Administration here and the National Institutes of Health, seem
more conservative. They suggest that medical treatment
often may be as effective as and perhaps more desirable
than surgery.

In addition, since bypass surgery is relatively new, studies giving long-term survival rates (twenty or more years)

are not yet available, so no one really knows for sure what the long-range outlook is.

Nonetheless, despite the spate of contradictory, conflicting and perplexing information, it is possible, through critical scrutiny of the studies, to learn facts that can be helpful to physicians and their patients in making decisions. And there are even a few areas of near agreement.

The first is that *bypass surgery is unquestionably successful in relieving pain.* Therefore, whatever the condition of the coronary arteries, a person who is in intractable pain from angina that cannot be helped medically should seriously consider the bypass operation.

Thirty-nine-year-old Melvin R. is an example. Melvin has been a foreman in a lumber mill for twenty years and has always been in good health, doing hard physical work. He swims twice a week, plays handball and exercises in the gym every Sunday. His blood pressure is normal, he is a few pounds underweight and he has a normal cholesterol level. His electrocardiogram is normal. In fact, his only risk factor is that he has been a three-pack-a-day smoker since he was seventeen.

Three months ago, Melvin began getting pains when he was lifting sheets of lumber. He tried to ignore them, but they continued to increase in intensity and frequency. Within a couple of weeks, he was often in pain throughout the day. Exercise and swimming were out of the question.

Cardiac catheterization revealed that Melvin had occlusions of more than 80 percent in his left anterior descending artery and in his circumflex artery. But his ejection fraction was a healthy 68 percent.

Since he had two-vessel disease, Melvin's doctor, a conservative practitioner, began by treating him with drugs. But Melvin could not get the kind of relief he needed to maintain his active life-style. He was unable to do his job and couldn't participate in the recreational activities that were so important to him.

When six more weeks passed with no change in his condition, Melvin and his physician agreed that coronary-bypass surgery was appropriate for him. As expected, because of Melvin's age and excellent physical condition, the operation went well and there were no complications. Within six weeks, Melvin was taking mile-long walks near his home and, two months later, returned to work. He has not experienced any recurrence of his incapacitating angina.

Betty C., a forty-year-old travel agent from Detroit, lives a more sedentary life than Melvin. She prefers to spend her free time reading and doing needlepoint. But Betty's family history is cluttered with victims of coronary artery disease. Her father, grandfather and uncle died as a result of heart attacks before they were thirty-five. Her mother has congestive heart failure, and her brother, who is fifty, has had two heart attacks. Betty, however, is in good health, except for nagging back problems which she has had since she fell from a ladder when she was twenty-five. Her cholesterol level is low-normal at 190; her blood pressure is 130/85, also normal; she is not diabetic and does not smoke. But a year ago she began to have chest pain when she vacuumed her rugs or walked quickly down the steps of her three-story house. When she rested, the pain subsided.

Her doctor prescribed medication, which seemed to help at first. But with time, the medicine was no longer effective. And the pains came more often. Sometimes they occurred even when Betty walked briskly to the corner grocery store.

In view of her ominous family history and her worsening symptoms, Betty's physician ordered a heart catheterization. It showed that Betty had two coronary arteries with significant blockages and another with a small, not yet significant, occlusion. Betty's ejection fraction was normal at 55 percent.

Betty felt strongly that she should have bypass surgery. So did her doctor, mainly because of her family background and because her pains were worsening. "Even though I am not a great athlete and live rather quietly, I didn't like the idea of being restricted and having to think three times before I did anything even slightly exertive," Betty says. "And I saw what happened to so many of my relatives. I was afraid *not* to have the surgery."

Like Melvin, Betty came through the operation successfully. She is back at work and experiencing no pain.

Betty and Melvin were "ideal" candidates for surgery. In fact, in an article titled "Surgical Treatment of Coronary Disease," a group from the Cleveland Clinic declared that the ideal patient—the one who can most benefit from bypass surgery—is significantly restricted by symptoms, has a significant amount of undamaged *myocardium* (heart muscle) jeopardized by coronary artery disease, but has diseased arteries that are large enough and free enough of distal disease (disease beyond the obstruction) to be treated with bypass graft.

Almost no physician would argue with a recommendation of coronary-bypass surgery when a patient is in good health but is experiencing symptoms that are disabling, is not responding to medication and is hampered in lifestyle.

Most studies show that coronary-bypass surgery is effective in relieving the pain associated with angina. A large percentage of patients undergoing the operation has total freedom from pain, and most others have at least partial relief. A number of studies support the premise that the quality of life is improved, at least at first, for as much as 90 percent of patients who have the operation. Often patients who were on a heavy medical regimen require less or no medication.

Forty-eight-year-old Wilma W., who lived on drugs for five years, has not taken any medication since her bypass surgery in 1978. "When I was convinced I didn't need them anymore, I had a pill-burning party," she says. "Actually, we didn't burn the pills . . . we just flushed them down the toilet and drank champagne to celebrate."

Dr. Willis Hurst reports that in surgical patients at Emory University Hospital in Atlanta, 92 percent have relief of symptoms and 62 percent are totally free of angina. And other studies indicate that long-term relief is obtained for a majority of patients. However, some research shows that the initial relief of pain after the operation is not always maintained. A study at Stanford University reported that after thirty months following surgery, 40 percent of patients were experiencing chest pain.

Relief from pain is not the only consideration. While it is true that patients who come to physicians do so because they are having disturbing and frightening symptoms, many doctors do not consider pain to be the most significant factor.

"It is not the symptoms a patient has, but where and how extensive the blockages are that should be the deciding factor when considering surgery," says Dr. Dudley Johnson. "It should be remembered that angina is a magnificent warning sign, when it occurs; but, unfortunately, it occurs too infrequently. Three-fourths of heart-attack victims have never had angina, but their coronary vessels were obviously in bad shape."

Forty-one-year-old Eleanor G. may be a case in point. Eleanor was a small, thin woman who operated a switchboard at a social-welfare agency. Her blood pressure was normal, as was her cholesterol level. There was no history of heart disease in her family. In fact, the only risk factors

Eleanor had were a history of heavy smoking and excessive stress. She was a single parent responsible for earning a living and taking care of a teenage daughter who was retarded. But she always seemed cheerful and insisted that she did not feel overburdened.

Her colleagues were stunned to learn one Saturday morning that their coworker had died of a heart attack the night before. She had been at work the day of her death, felt well and had no complaints. At home, she talked of feeling slightly nauseous and went to bed early. Three hours later, she suffered severe chest pain that led to "sudden death."

Whether or not surgery can protect a person from sudden death (when he or she, unlike Eleanor, is fortunate enough to have symptoms indicating that something is wrong) or heart attack is still an unsettled issue. In an article entitled "The First Decade of Aortocoronary Bypass Grafting—1967–1977," published in *Circulation*, the official journal of the American Heart Association, Drs. Henry D. McIntosh and Jorge A. Garcia maintain that "there are, at present, no conclusive data in the literature to support the concept that aortocoronary bypass graft is superior to adequate medical management to prevent or even ameliorate other signs and symptoms of ischemic heart disease (a condition caused by clogged coronary arteries resulting in poor blood flow to the heart) such as myocardial infarction or heart failure. The procedure is, therefore, not recommended for these purposes. There are also inadequate data to support the thesis that aortocoronary bypass grafting prevents the occurrence of 'sudden death' better than intensive medical therapy."

However, Dr. Floyd Loop of the Cleveland Clinic says that McIntosh and Garcia's statement is no longer valid. He cites the influence of coronary bypass on the incidence of late postoperative heart attack (occurring more than thirty days after surgery), based on a study of 2,224 patients, 80 percent of whom had multiple-vessel obstruction. After an average follow-up of two and a half years, the yearly rate of heart attack averaged 2.1 percent, of which 29 percent was fatal. This yielded an annual 0.6 percent rate of fatal heart attack in persons who had undergone surgery.

This group of patients was compared with a ten-year study of the natural history of patients with ischemic heart disease. The rate of heart attack here was 6 percent annually, and a 3.7 percent annual death rate from heart attack was reported.

And a report from the Angiography Registry of Seattle Heart Watch concludes that "saphenous vein bypass grafting appears to reduce cardiac death rates in patients with two-vessel disease; this is due to a reduction in sudden cardiac deaths."

Dr. McIntosh agrees that "since the manuscript [the one referred to earlier] was written, there has been a gratifying reduction in the operative mortality for bypass surgery in most centers and, indeed, there has been a striking reduction in the incidence of perioperative myocardial infarctions [heart attacks during the hospital stay]. In addition there has been reasonably good evidence that bypass surgery will prolong life in patients who are symptomatic and who have significant stenosis [blockages] of the left main coronary artery or significant stenosis of the three major vessels of the coronary arteries. As life is prolonged in such patients, indeed sudden death may be postponed in patients who are operated . . . ."

Still, he maintains that medical management of coronary patients has improved dramatically also and that "we really don't know what the incidence of fatal heart attacks is in patients who are treated nonoperatively by current medical methods, which include reduction of risk factors, appropriate medications and changes in lifestyle."

Because certain clogged arteries are more worrisome than others, the location and extent of blockages may count heavily in determining who is a candidate for surgery.

Left Main Coronary Artery

If a person's blockage, as shown on a coronary angiogram, is in the left main coronary artery, it is critical; that artery is the main supplier of blood to the left ventricle, which in turn furnishes blood to the entire body. In this case, almost everyone agrees that surgery should be done.

"Almost half of these people will die within five years if they are not bypassed," says Deborah Hospital's Dr. Gerald Lemole, who performed the first coronary bypass done in Pennsylvania in 1969, "So there is no question that for these people [who comprise about 10 percent of all persons with coronary artery disease], surgery is a must."

Studies support Dr. Lemole. The Veterans Administration Cooperative Study (see Appendix), one of the largest ever done to compare results of surgically and medically treated patients, revealed that 36 percent of patients with left main disease who were not operated on were dead at four years of follow-up. And a recently published study from the Montreal Heart Institute and Participating CASS (Coronary Artery Surgery Study) Sites, which looked at 1,492 patients with left main coronary disease, shows significantly improved survival for patients who received bypass.

Patients came from fifteen hospitals—the University of Alabama in Birmingham, Albany Medical College, Boston University, Marshfield Medical Foundation, Massachusetts General Hospital, Montreal Heart Institute, New York University School of Medicine, St. Louis School of Medicine, Stanford University, Yale University, Loma

Linda University, Mayo Clinic, Medical College of Wisconsin, Miami Heart Institute and St. Luke's Hospital Center. The study was coordinated at the University of Washington in Seattle and was funded by the National Heart, Lung, and Blood Institute.

There were two groups of patients: 1,183 who had bypass surgery and 309 who received medical care and did not go to the operating room. Both groups were alike in terms of age, gender, history of previous heart attacks, frequency of coronary risk factors (such as extent of smoking) and extent of coronary artery disease. The group that went to surgery, however, tended to have more severe symptoms and often needed more medication before surgery to maintain control. This group also had more severe left main disease (more extensive narrowing of vessels), but their left ventricles tended to perform better than those of the medical group.

Four years after surgery, eighty-eight percent of the group that had been operated on was alive, as compared to only 63 percent of the group treated medically. Younger patients did better than older patients, but in every age category the four-year survival for the surgical patients was better. The older patients who did not undergo surgery had a poor prognosis, with only 51 percent alive four years later, compared to 82 percent of those who had had surgery.

The function of the left ventricle was crucial (because the ventricle pumps blood through the body), and the survival rates correlate with its degree of impairment. In the operative group, the three-year survival rate in patients with good left ventricular function was 95 percent, compared to 75 percent for those with poor ventricular function. In the medical group, patients with good left ventricles had an 84 percent survival rate at the end of three years, but only 46 percent of those with poor left ventricles were alive after thirty-six months.

However, even among patients with disease of the left main coronary artery, where surgery is generally recommended, there are subsets of patients who are less likely than others to benefit from an operation.

For instance, consider patients whose circulation is dominated by the right side of the heart or whose circulation is evenly balanced between the left and right sides of the heart (90 percent of all people have right-dominated circulation, a determination which is made at catheterization). When patients with left main disease but normal left ventricles had blockages of more than 50 percent in the right coronary artery, surgery significantly improved survival. But when the right coronary artery had a blockage, less than 50 percent, surgery did not improve survival rates. It was encouraging that the three-year survival of patients with left main coronary disease who did not receive surgery was as high as 85 percent when they had three characteristics:

- Circulation dominated by the right coronary artery or balanced circulation;
- A blockage of less than 50 percent in the right coronary artery;
- Normal left ventricular function.

Bypass surgery *did not* improve survival in left main disease patients with a left dominant circulation, mainly because the operative mortality in this group was a whopping 10 percent.

Since long-term survival is affected by many factors other than presence of disease in the left main coronary artery, the CASS study divided patients into four groups by estimated risk. The risk factors were considered in order of importance: choice of therapy (the most important determinant of survival; most studies indicate that patients with left main disease are at significantly higher risk if they do not have the bypass operation); left ventricular score (the function of the left ventricle); heart failure score (the presence and extent of heart failure); age; percent of the blockage of the left main artery; coronary dominance (which artery dominates circulation); hypertension; and more than 50 percent blockage of a *dominant* right coronary artery. The study showed that survival was better for the surgical patients, no matter the risk group. But the impact of surgery on survival was definitely greater for patients with the highest risks.

The CASS investigators concluded that bypass surgery "prolongs life in most patients with left main coronary disease, especially those with severe left main coronary narrowing or impaired left ventricular function. In nonoperated patients with left main disease, the most important determinants of survival are the percent of left main stenosis [blockage], left ventricular function, severity of angina, age and hypertension. In patients who undergo surgery, the most important determinants of long-term survival are preoperative left ventricular function and age."

Another study from Duke University Medical Center showed that patients with left main disease identified as "low-risk" had a three-year survival rate of only 74 percent without surgery. And patients with left main disease but normal ventricular function, studied at the Cleveland Clinic, had a five-year survival rate of only 55 percent if they did not have surgery. In both of these studies, the annual mortality rate was 9 percent.

A study done at the University of Alabama Medical Center between 1966 and 1975 included 179 patients with disease of the left main coronary artery. Thirty-eight were treated medically, and 149 underwent bypass surgery. At the end of one year, 89 percent of the surgical group was alive, but only 73 percent of the medical group survived. At twenty-four months, 86 percent of the surgical patients were alive, as compared to only 65 percent of those treated medically. The investigators in this study, headed by Dr. Albert Oberman, suggest that it is usually difficult to compare surgically and medically treated patients without randomizing them because of the bias in selecting patients for each group. However, in this study, only patients who were considered to be surgical candidates, but who were treated medically instead, were considered.

The Veterans Administration Cooperative Group for the Study of Surgery for Coronary Arterial Occlusive Disease, the most important major randomized study in the field (see Appendix), published the results of its investigation of a subgroup of patients with disease of the left main coronary artery. Included were 113 patients from 13 hospitals, 53 of whom had been randomly allocated to medical treatment and 60 to surgery. The study took place from January 1970 through December 1974.

All patients were male, and all had had angina for at least six months. Arteriography indicated that all would be suitable candidates for bypass surgery. In addition to the obstruction which was shown on an angiograph, all of the men had significant disabling angina pectoris, and their electrocardiograms (exercise or resting) showed abnormalities consistent with atherosclerosis. The average age of patients in the medical group was fifty-four; in the surgical group, fifty-two.

Both groups were evenly matched for risk factors. For example, 73.6 percent of the medical group was free of hypertension, as was 75 percent of the surgical group. History of a heart attack was present in 45.3 percent of the medical patients and 46.7 percent of the surgical patients. Other variables which correlated in both groups included the duration of angina; history of coronary heart failure, stroke or diabetes; or family history of coronary disease. Approximately 62 percent of all patients (medical and surgical) were in Class II or IV of the New York Heart Association Functional Classification (see Chapter 1).

No patient had total blockage of the left main coronary artery (blockages ranged from 50 percent to 90 percent), but 62 percent of those treated medically had significant blockages of the left anterior descending, circumflex and right coronary arteries, in addition to the left main occlusion. Fifty-three percent of surgical patients had similar blockages. Only one surgical patient had disease confined to the left main coronary artery. Fifteen medical patients and seventeen surgical patients had blockages of more than 90 percent in the left main artery.

Patients were grouped into those with an ejection fraction of 50 percent or more (healthy), or less than 50 percent (not as favorable). The high-risk group among the total population of 113 patients included those with left main disease, plus disease of the right coronary artery, plus a poor ejection fraction.

Follow-up studies were made every three months for the first two years, at which time the degree of angina experienced by the patient was recorded and an electrocardiogram (sometimes a stress test) was taken. Most patients who underwent surgery also had arteriography at the end of the first year to determine whether their grafts were open.

Of the original 113 patients, one in the surgical group and six in the medical group did not follow the therapy prescribed. Two who had been assigned to medical care died within one month.

Of the fifty-nine patients who had surgery, 14 percent died during the operation or within thirty days afterwards. In the study's first two years, there were five operative deaths in twenty patients, but in the last three years, this was reduced to 7 percent in forty-five operated cases.

Of patients who were randomized in the last three years of the study, twelve of forty-one medical patients (20 percent) died. Only three of forty-two surgical patients (7 percent) did not survive. It is important to note that survival curves for the patients who were randomized early in the program (from 1970–1971) were not statistically different at any stage of the follow-up period. But of the eighty-three patients who entered the study later (when the operative mortality decreased), the difference in survival between the two groups—the surgical group surviving longer—was significant.

The patients were also considered in terms of the way they were grouped—those with good and poor ejection fractions. Patients with normal ejection fractions showed little difference in the survival curve between medical and surgical groups. For instance, of thirty-six patients with good ejection fractions, there were five deaths in those treated medically and two in those treated surgically. However, in the group with the poor ejection fraction, there were fourteen medical and nine surgical deaths.

The investigations concluded that "the cumulative survival rate of surgically randomized patients [with left main disease] was significantly better statistically than medically randomized patients, when the survival rates were compared at eighteen, twenty-four and thirty months following entry into the study. At thirty-six months, with the late deaths of two surgical patients, the difference between the two groups decreased."

But while most practitioners have concluded that surgery will improve the outlook for patients with left main disease, there are a few who are uncertain that medical treatment is not equally effective for some patients.

Dr. Philip J. Podrid, research associate at Harvard School of Public Health and associate in medicine at

Brigham and Women's Hospital in Boston, does not feel that surgery is necessary in all patients with disease of the left main coronary artery. He explains that few people have left main disease without other vessels also being involved. In these cases, he says, the patient will usually have a lot of angina and may need an operation if the symptoms cannot be controlled medically. But if she or he can be managed with drugs and life-style changes, there is no reason to have surgery even if the left main coronary artery is blocked. There is no evidence, he says, to demonstrate that life will be prolonged or the risk of heart attack will be diminished if surgery is performed in patients who do not have symptoms.

It may depend on other factors, says Dr. R. J. Sung in a paper published in *Circulation* magazine. "It may be that the mortality is extremely high in these [left main] patients with poor distal vessels technically unsuitable for surgery [distal vessels are branches of main arteries that are smaller and often more difficult to bypass]. On the other hand, mortality is relatively low in patients who have technically bypassable lesions, whether treated surgically or medically. Surgery does appear, however, to be more effective in providing symptomatic and clinical improvement . . . it appears doubtful that angiographic evidence of left main coronary obstruction alone justifies surgical therapy."

Dr. Stephen E. Epstein, chief of the Cardiology Branch of the National Heart, Lung, and Blood Institute of the National Institutes of Health, comments that while all of the studies performed on persons with left main disease included only highly symptomatic subjects (and results could be different with subjects less symptomatic), "the left main coronary artery patient is unique in the extent of myocardium jeopardized and the paucity of opportunity for the development of compensatory collateral blood flow. The rapid progression of such lesions might be expected to produce a relatively high incidence of catastrophic events in patients with few antecedent symptoms. These considerations represent the principal justification for identifying and promptly operating on significant lesions of the left main artery in patients with coronary artery disease who lack severe symptoms. . . ."

In summary, the *only two conditions* about which there is almost universal agreement that surgery is the treatment of choice are:

1. The patient with incapacitating angina that cannot be relieved by *appropiate* medical management. In these cases, relief of pain is the major reason for the operation, and there is agreement that bypass surgery is effective in providing it.
2. The patient with disease of the left main coronary artery because the blood supply to the critical left ventricle is compromised. In such situations, many but not all studies have shown that the mortality rate without surgery is excessively high.

For all other patients with coronary artery disease, the decision depends largely on whom you ask, which studies you choose to believe and what seems to make sense for a specific person.

What makes sense depends on a number of factors. Most important, perhaps, is the *extent of the disease*— which vessels are blocked and how significant the blockages are.

The *condition of the patient's left ventricle* is critical and often figures heavily in determining not only his prognosis with or without surgery, but how great his risk would be if he had an operation.

Consideration must be given, too, to the nature of the patient's angina. Is it stable, unstable or preinfarction (so serious that it may indicate an oncoming heart attack) angina? Is it responding to medical treatment? What is causing it? Is there history of a heart attack? What are the patient's risk factors, such as hypertension, age, sex, cholesterol level, history of congestive heart failure? What about the patient who has no symptoms, but who knows, because he has had an angiogram, that he has significant blockages? Let us explore each aspect.

Once it is known that a patient *does not have* disease of his left main coronary artery (only 10 percent of patients do), it is important to know, through angiography, how many vessels are blocked, which ones they are and what the percentage of obstruction is. For instance, a person may have blockages in one, two or all three of his coronary vessels.

Narrowing of less than 50 percent in any artery would not usually constitute a blockage significant enough to require surgery because it does not compromise the maximum flow of blood from the heart. Persons with obstructions of 50 to 60 percent will experience only mild restriction of blood flow, probably when they are exercising or under stress. However, when blockages exceed 85 percent, blood flow while a patient is at rest is likely to become impaired.

Dr. Donald Miller, Jr., of Seattle, in his book, *The Practice of Coronary Artery Bypass Surgery,* says that patients with lesions of 50 to 60 percent will have a blood flow that is only minimally restricted, little physical disability and a low risk of death from heart disease or heart attack. But patients with blockages of 85 percent or greater have often already had a heart attack and are at higher risk.

Triple Vessel Disease

When there is significant disease of all *three major vessels,* as shown on an angiogram, many studies suggest that surgery will prolong life. One of the most prominent research projects is the European Cooperative Study, in which investigators from twelve European countries participated; included were 768 men under sixty-five with angina, all with good "ejection fractions." Three hundred seventy-three patients were allotted to medical and 395 to surgical treatment between 1973 and 1976. All had had angina pectoris for more than three months, and all of the angiograms demonstrated lesions of more than 50 percent in at least two coronary arteries.

Patients with obstruction in the left main coronary artery were included in some of the participating centers. The patients in each group had similar risk factors. For instance, 43 percent of those in the medical and surgical groups were smokers; 15 percent of those in the medical group and 18 percent of those in the surgical group had hypertension.

Of the 373 patients who were treated medically, 188 had three-vessel disease. Two hundred nineteen of the surgically treated patients had disease of three vessels. At the end of two years, the survival rate of the surgical patients was 95.9 percent; of the medical patients, it was 89.9 percent, a significant difference.

However, the major study of the Veterans Administration, which looked at 1,015 patients, indicated that there was no statistically significant difference in survival between the patients in that group who had triple-vessel disease, whether they were treated medically or surgically. But this study has been soundly criticized by some physicians and surgeons, and there are other studies that yield contradictory findings (see Appendix). In addition, follow-up research on patients entered into the original Veterans Administration study (reported in *Circulation* in July 1981) suggests that there may be certain subsets of patients with triple-vessel disease who would be more likely to benefit from surgery. These are patients who, in addition to having triple-vessel disease, have several of the following risk factors: severe angina, an abnormal electrocardiogram at rest, a history of heart attack and the presence of hypertension.

Another startling study, published November 5, 1981 in the New England Journal of Medicine (see Appendix I), provides more evidence that medical rather than surgical treatment may be effective for many patients with multivessel (two or three vessel) disease. The study followed, for an average of 59 months, 142 men who had demonstrated profound ST-segment depression on their electrocardiographs during stress testing. This is a finding that has been associated with severe multivessel disease. Traditionally, persons who demonstrate this ST depression are sent for coronary angiograms and possibly for bypass surgery. Now, the authors of the study say that "bypass surgery is rarely necessary for these patients." They report that medical management is highly sucessful and is associated with a low mortality. Their mortality rate was 1.4 percent a year.

Nonetheless, Emory's Dr. Hurst makes a strong case for the improved survival of persons with triple-vessel disease after surgery. In his analysis, based on the examination of studies conducted at leading medical centers, he concludes that the long-term survival of patients with triple-vessel disease who undergo coronary bypass surgery is dramatically improved over patients who do not have the operation.

Dr. Hurst cites a five-year survival curve of 740 patients who had bypass surgery at the Buffalo General Hospital. The survival rate is about 88 percent at five years in the group treated by surgery, compared with 48 to 58 percent in medically treated patients. Reports from the Peter Bent Brigham Hospital in Boston indicate a survival rate of 97 percent at five years in patients who had bypass surgery for triple-vessel disease, compared to a 56 percent cumulative survival rate at four years in a group of patients treated medically at the Cleveland Clinic. Dr. N. T. Kouchoukos reported on a group of patients followed at the University of Alabama in Birmingham. The patients were not randomized, but they were treated and studied during the same time period. At forty-six months, 83 percent of the surgical group, but only 53 percent of the medical group (consisting of patients who were candidates for surgery but who did not have the operation), were alive. And Drs. Michael DeBakey and Gerald Lawrie at the Baylor College of Medicine say that more than fourteen years of follow-up on patients has convinced them that patients with good ventricular function can expect a normal survival rate after operation.

Nonetheless, the National Institutes of Health's Dr. Stephen Epstein points out that groups not randomized can produce critically different outcomes than those that are randomized, because selection factors (who goes into which group) have a powerful influence over results. He also says that patients treated medically who were reported on in earlier years cannot be used as a control group for patients receiving surgery (which was the case in many studies) because medical treatment is dramatically different today. And he says that "virtually all published natural history studies of patients [the history of patients who do not have surgical intervention] with angiographically documented coronary artery disease are derived from large medical centers to which more seriously symptomatic patients are usually referred." Dr. Epstein believes that the course of the disease and the prognosis are often different in patients who have symptoms and patients who do not.

Double- and Single-Vessel Disease

The treatment course for persons with disease of one or two vessels is one of the most controversial issues in medicine. Wisconsin's Dr. Dudley Johnson says he would operate on anyone with significant disease of one vessel because "it makes sense that if you improve the flow of blood to the heart, the patient's chances of survival improve too."

On the other hand, many doctors are convinced that patients with single-vessel and perhaps even double-vessel disease can do just as well if they are treated medically, and that surgery, in fact, does not prolong life.

An exception would be left main disease or a lesion located close to the origin of the left anterior descending artery, because an obstruction there could effectively close off much of the blood supply to the left ventricle.

The European Collaborative Randomized Trial, in fact, found no significant difference in the three- to five-year survival rates for medical and surgical patients with two-vessel disease. Medical patients with no obstructions in the left anterior descending artery had a 96 percent survival rate at sixty months; those whose LADs were blocked had a survival rate of 82 percent.

And a consensus statement by the National Institutes of Health, issued in December 1980, states that "the two large randomized studies (the European study and the Veterans Administration study) do not provide evidence of improved survival after surgery in patients with two-vessel disease, regardless of the status of the left ventricle. But some observational studies have suggested improvement in survival after surgery of patients with two-vessel disease and moderate impairment of left ventricular function.

"There is no evidence of improved survival after surgery in patients with single-vessel disease, regardless of left ventricular functional status." (Chairman of the consensus committee was Dr. Robert L. Frye, chairman of the division of cardiovascular diseases at the Mayo Clinic.)

Types of Angina

Despite the number of vessels that may be involved, there is a difference in the way many doctors will treat stable angina and angina considered "unstable." *Stable angina* is described as anginal pain that has persisted for a long period—six months or more—unchanged in intensity and controlled by medication. For this condition, a majority of physicians would not perform surgery unless there was evidence of left main disease or significant triple-vessel disease. "A man who has had angina for five years, who responds to medication and has had no increase of symptoms, would be considered stable," says Emory's Dr. Hurst. "His situation is less threatening than the man with new angina, but some of these patients need surgery."

Peter T., for instance, had his first angina symptom fifteen years ago when he was sixty, and just before bypass surgery was common.

"I didn't understand it," Peter says. "I had never been sick a day in my life. The only time I was in a hospital was to have my wisdom teeth pulled when I was twenty-two. I didn't like these pains I was getting in my chest. They slowed me down."

Peter's doctor, a general practitioner, prescribed nitroglycerin, which he instructed him to place under his tongue whenever the angina came. Peter has been using nitroglycerin since that time. The frequency and intensity of his pain has not changed, and his electrocardiogram, which is taken every six months, is normal.

His condition would be considered stable, and none but the most aggressive physician would suggest surgery. (Dr. Hurst suggests that it is not possible to know with certainty that Peter is indeed suffering from coronary atherosclerosis because he has not been tested.)

Preinfarction or "crescendo" angina patients would be considered surgical candidates by many physicians. Their condition is characterized by persistent pain unrelieved by medication, lasting more than a half-hour and accompanied by electrocardiographic changes showing lack of blood to the heart muscle. These are the patients who are usually hospitalized so their angina can be brought under control and a heart attack avoided.

"I think that anyone with preinfarction angina would be a candidate for surgery, especially if a critical vessel is involved," says Dr. Denton Cooley, one of the country's leading heart surgeons.

Mildred S., a seventy-two-year-old woman who has had stable angina for ten years, was almost strangled one night by piercing pain that she could not control with her customary medication. Her cardiologist, whom she called at two A.M., met her at the hospital and prescribed aggressive medication to stabilize her condition. Four days later, Mildred had a heart catheterization which showed a 95-percent blockage of the left main coronary artery.

"I think you're going to be OK if you have surgery," her doctor, who was a longtime friend, told her. "But it is risky because of your age and the location of your blockage."

Mildred responded, "I would rather die on the operating table trying to help myself live than walk around living, waiting to drop dead anytime."

The operation was performed immediately . . . and was a success. Six days later, Mildred was strolling through the corridors of the hospital and insisting that she had to go home. It was spring-planting time, and she didn't want to miss the tulips.

Patients with *unstable angina* are a source of additional conflict, partly because so many kinds of symptoms are lumped into this category. They include:

- People who have intense and prolonged angina while resting, with little or no response to medication;
- People who have had angina with activity, whose discomfort has increased in frequency and intensity during the past three months;
- Patients who experience angina within thirty days after a heart attack;
- Anyone with new angina.

Here, the coronary anatomy (as determined by a heart catheterization) and the discomfort of the patient are determining.

"It is an individual decision that must be tailored to each patient based on the results of his catheterization and his symptoms," says Dr. Paul Walinsky, a cardiologist at Jefferson Medical College in Philadelphia. "If the blockage, for instance, is 70 percent and the patient can control symptoms with medication, there would be less indication for surgery than a patient with a 95 percent obstruction."

On the other hand, if the same patient were experiencing intractable pain despite appropriate medication, and he had to decrease his activity and disliked doing so, he might choose surgery.

Dr. C. Richard Conti of the Division of Cardiovascular Medicine at the University of Florida says that recent studies show that patients with unstable angina can benefit from appropriate medical management, which includes hospitalization, the use of medication, bed rest and sedation. In an article he wrote for *Cardiovascular Reviews and Reports* he says, "Recent studies show that with appropriate medical management . . . most patients will have relief of angina and will neither proceed to myocardial infarction [heart attack] nor die."

Because of conflicting views on patients with unstable angina, the National Heart, Lung, and Blood Institute undertook a study in which such patients were randomized either to surgical or nonsurgical therapy. Results demonstrated no advantage for those who were operated on with respect to early death or heart attack (see Appendix). Dr. Conti, therefore, believes that patients with unstable angina should be given intensive medical therapy and that surgery should be considered only if the patient is not relieved of pain. All patients should have coronary angiography, and if the patient has severe left main coronary artery disease (as evidenced on the angiogram), or poor performance on stress testing with disease of several vessels, he feels that surgery is warranted.

History of Heart Attack

What about the person who has already had a heart attack? Is she or he a candidate for bypass surgery? It depends. Approximately 10 to 15 percent of all patients die in the first year following heart attack. What makes them different from the 85 to 90 percent who survive the first twelve months?

A critical yardstick is their "ejection fraction," which reveals the state of the left ventricle. If the "ejection fraction" (see Chapter 3) is less than 40 percent at the time of discharge from the hospital, the prognosis is poor. Eighty-five percent of these patients do not make it through the first year following the myocardial infarction. (Tests, described in Chapter 3, can measure ejection fraction.)

Another indicator that a person who has suffered a heart attack may be in danger is evidence of significant changes on an electrocardiogram demonstrated while exercising.

For these high-risk patients, bypass surgery should be considered.

A Philadelphia psychologist, Melvin F., who suffered a heart attack when he was thirty-seven, has refused to have a heart catheterization, even though his cardiologist has urged him to do so. The physician feels it is important, in view of Melvin's history (a father who died at forty-five of heart disease and a brother with angina), to learn which arteries are blocked and to what extent. But Melvin has a good ejection fraction (75 percent) and a negative stress test. He goes skiing every weekend in the winter, scuba diving every weekend in the summer, paints his house and mows his lawn. Another cardiologist has told him that, based on his ejection fraction and his tolerance to exercise, he is not, at present, a candidate for catheterization or surgery.

The type of angina and history of a heart attack are not the only factors that influence who will benefit from surgery and who will not. There are other critical considerations. Many of them are unfamiliar to patients who are unaware, in fact, of important information about themselves that could bear on a thoughtful decision between surgery and medical care.

One of the most significant is:

The condition of the left ventricle. A healthy left ventricle indicates that the pumping mechanism of the heart is effective and able to do its job of supplying the body with blood. There are several ways to test for ventricular function. One is checking the ejection fraction (discussed in Chapter 3), which can be done through noninvasive ventriculograms or during catheterization. No matter the degree of blockage, patients with good ejection fractions can be expected to do better than patients with poor ones. This is true whether they are treated medically or surgically.

The Seattle Heart Watch, a cooperative, community-wide registry, its major goal to identify people at risk of sudden cardiac death, analyzed 746 medically treated patients who had arteriography for suspected coronary disease between January 1, 1971, and December 31, 1974, and 1,870 patients who had heart-bypass surgery between January 1, 1969, and December 31, 1974. The study found that, for medically treated patients, the ejection fraction was the factor most predictive of survival. With surgically treated patients, ejection fraction was the second most predictive factor. The first was ventricular arrhythmia on a resting electrocardiogram, which, if present, compromised survival.

An exception may be a patient such as fifty-two-year-old Roger A. He has disease of three coronary arteries but has no symptoms and an ejection fraction of 40, a little subnormal. (Roger's coronary-artery blockages were revealed when a mandatory stress test given by his employer turned out to be positive. He then underwent catheterization.) "With patients who have no symptoms or only mild symptoms, the ejection fraction, as long as it is more than 20, doesn't seem to be as powerful a predictor of the patient's outcome as it is when patients have angina," says National Institutes of Health's Dr. Stephen Epstein. Roger has been advised to have surgery but is unwilling because he feels so well.

Another yardstick to check the left ventricular function is called the *end-diastolic pressure,* a measurement that can be taken only during catheterization, with the catheter inserted in the left ventricle. This refers to the pressure at the end of the diastolic phase of heart pumping when the heart is most relaxed. Normal end-diastolic pressure would be about 10 or 12. A higher reading means that the heart does not have much reserve, cannot handle the fluid produced by the blood, and that damage to the ventricle is high.

Many physicians consider the ejection fraction to be a better predictor of the function of the left ventricle than the end-diastolic pressure, because the latter is variable. If you add fluid, it will rise. A rule of thumb, says cardiac surgeon Dr. Gerald Lemole, is that when the end-diastolic pressure is higher than the ejection fraction, it means that the heart muscle is functioning poorly, that the person is not a good candidate for surgery. And it is known that bypass surgery cannot restore dead heart muscle.

"However, sometimes the heart muscle just seems dead but is not," says Dr. Richard Helfant of the University of Pennsylvania. "It is just not contracting normally because the oxygen supply to it is so seriously impaired." This heart muscle is what he and Dr. Lemole call "scared stiff" but has the potential for improving.

Dr. Helfant can differentiate between the two. First, he gives the patient a traditional heart catheterization (described in Chapter 3) in order to see the impaired heart muscle. Then the patient puts a nitroglycerin tablet under his tongue to create a better balance between the oxygen needs of the heart muscle and the supply available to it. This permits the muscle to increase its ability to contract if it is capable. A repeat angiogram a few minutes later shows the effect on the heart muscle.

"If there is improvement, it indicates that bypass surgery, which increases oxygen supply, would have the same effect," says Dr. Helfant. "Indeed, we have seen that it does. When we re-evaluate patients after surgery, we are astounded, in these cases, at the restored heart muscle."

It is not yet known what effect surgery would have on the prognosis of such patients, but it is reasonable to assume that the incidence of mortality would be reduced, especially if left main or triple-vessel disease is present.

The Cause of the Angina

While constricted arteries are often the cause of angina, there can be another reason, and it is crucial that the cause of the pain be determined before a decision about surgery is made. Dr. Attilio Maseri, a professor at the University of London's Royal Postgraduate Medical School, says that while there is no question that narrowed arteries eventually block blood flow to the heart and cause some heart attacks, there is also evidence of "another major culprit"—spasms that temporarily constrict vessels that are not—or are only partially—clogged.

"These constrictions of arteries supplying blood to the heart can cause sudden death or heart attacks by closing down the blood supply, just as effectively as can the narrowed arteries," says Dr. Maseri. One aspect of this phenomenon is known as *Prinzmetal's variant angina*, named for Dr. Myron Prinzmetal, a Los Angeles cardiologist who described the syndrome in the late 1940s.

Doctors can distinguish what is causing a person's chest pains—clogged arteries or spasms—by taking a detailed medical history, Dr. Maseri insists. He says that people who consistently experience chest pain at a given level of exercise or stress are probably suffering from critical blockage in their arteries. But those whose pain is often not related to exercise probably have artery constriction from time to time.

There seem to be two distinct groups of persons who have Prinzmetal's variant angina. One group has coronary artery spasm superimposed on blockage of the coronary arteries. These patients often have chest pain with exertion, at first, and later experience chest discomfort at rest. They also have a frequent history of heart attack.

The second group has coronary artery spasm without underlying coronary artery disease, and they usually do not have angina at rest; nor do they have a history of myocardial infarction. The attacks of angina tend to be cyclical; that is, the attacks will appear at the same time each day and may be present for several days or several weeks, then vanish for a time and begin again. If patients receive an electrocardiogram during an attack, there will usually be transient elevations of the ST segment. This differs from classic angina patients whose electrocardiograms will show ST segment depressions.

Many studies have shown that patients who suffer with Prinzmetal's angina unaccompanied by coronary artery disease will probably not be helped by bypass surgery.

Joel T., fifty-one, is a case in point. He had been suffering from chest pain atypical of angina. It usually came on at the same time each day, often when he was lying in bed, reading a magazine or watching television. Sometimes an attack occurred during a meeting when he was not agitated and just sitting quietly.

His electrocardiogram showed elevation in the ST segment, often indicative of variant angina. But subsequent catheterization revealed two-vessel disease, blockage of 80 and 70 percent, for which surgery was recommended. Joel had a good ejection fraction (which he didn't know at the time) and was told that he was an ideal surgical candidate.

"I believed that the operation would take my pain away," Joel recalls. "And I really wasn't afraid. So many people were having it. It seemed to be more common than gall bladder operations or appendectomies."

The operation went smoothly, and Joel recovered without incident. But less than a month later, his old chest pains returned. After that, they recurred even more frequently and with more intensity than they had before the surgery.

"The doctors began to say something about the cause of my angina being twofold," Joel says. "That was the first time I ever heard anything about spasm being responsible for my pain as well as the blocked arteries. I was really angry. I had gone through a useless operation, taken time off from work, been away from my family, had two incisions [leg and chest] to show for my trouble, and I was worse off than I had been before.

"It is outrageous that no one told me that my angina was different—and that the chances of an operation helping me were not as great as if I had only blocked arteries. I think I would have made a different choice. Now I feel that my body has been abused and my intelligence has been insulted. I feel like somebody's experiment."

Age of Patient

It is uniformly acknowledged that age is an important factor in determining a candidate for surgery. Often, a person's age will correlate to the level of activity with which he is satisfied; a man of seventy-five who is content to live a sedentary life may be able to tolerate his angina, while a younger person accustomed to an action-packed existence might want surgery because he cannot live comfortably with his symptoms.

Consider, for instance, seventy-two-year-old Minnie M. Minnie has had angina for the past four years, which has increased in intensity and frequency but has not been incapacitating. "I know I can't do all of the things I used to do," Minnie says. "But I'm content to be a little quieter now. I am retired, and I keep myself busy knitting and sewing dresses for my granddaughter. I can't walk too far because I get out of breath, but one has to expect those things when you get older. I don't mind. I always say, 'As long as I can get out of bed in the morning and take care of my family [Minnie has a husband and a sister who live with her] and my house, I am thankful.' I don't want an operation. I'm too old for that sort of thing."

Other men and women Minnie's age or older, however, are not willing to settle for less just because they have reached their seventh decade. Seventy-four-year-old Max J. still wants to swim every day. Roman S., who is seventy-five, likes to ride his bicycle several miles a week. Shirley R., seventy-one, and her husband, Harry, seventy-six, don't want to give up the square dancing they do twice a week.

Doctors, therefore, have had to look carefully at the surgical risks and results with persons who need and want bypass operations to keep up with their youth.

In the early days of bypass surgery, the mortality rate of older persons was considerably higher than that of younger ones. But recent advances are responsible for the operation being offered as an alternative to those who are in the seventh decade of life. A study from the Division of Surgery of the Texas Heart Institute of St. Luke's Episcopal and Texas Children's Hospitals in Houston reports on ninety-five patients, seventy or older, who had bypass surgery between November 1969 and June 1974. Twenty-one of the patients had valve problems in addition to blocked arteries, and a left ventricular *aneurysm* (a scarred area of the heart which can hold a lot of blood) was present in seven. During the first six months of 1974, the mortality rate of twenty-one older patients was only 4.8 percent, compared with an overall mortality rate of 22.1 percent in earlier years. It is important, say the study's authors, that patients have coronary artery surgery before they have suffered irreversible heart damage from repeated heart attacks, all of which makes them riskier surgical candidates.

There has been as much concern about the benefits of coronary artery surgery for patients younger than forty. But a report from Texas, which analyzed seventy-three patients between twenty-eight and thirty-eight, found that the results seem to justify surgery. Surgical mortality was 5.5 percent, and improvement in symptoms (incapacitating or preinfarction angina were present in 94.5 percent before the operation) occurred in 96 percent. Angiograms taken after surgery showed that 79 percent of the grafts were open.

The Nature of the Disease

Many physicians are pessimistic about the success of surgery when the disease is too widespread and involves many small, difficult-to-bypass coronary branches.

Sometimes there are patients who choose surgery but have been turned down because their disease is too diffuse, because too many tiny distal vessels are involved or because they have a poor left ventricular function. These patients are often told that they are inoperable.

But Wisconsin's Dr. Johnson disagrees. "During the last ten years, I have never denied a patient surgery because of diffuse disease, providing his ventricular function [the ability of the heart to pump blood into the body] was satisfactory [greater than 30 percent].

"The major problem is not in deciding who is a candidate for surgery, but in defining the ability of a surgeon to handle patients who may have widespread disease in secondary small coronary branches, a condition which sometimes involves five to eight bypasses. Some surgeons can and do handle small vessels with good results. Others cannot."

This means that Dr. Johnson has had to bypass many secondary small coronary branches and that he has often inserted five to eight grafts, more than many heart surgeons are willing to do. While it is known that grafts to those smaller secondary vessels have a greater chance of closing, Dr. Johnson's success rate has been high. In a group of patients operated on from 1970 through 1975, with normal ventricular function but diffuse disease requiring four to eight grafts, his mortality rate has been 0.86 a year, slightly less than the mortality rate for the general population in a similar age group.

Dr. Johnson will also operate on patients with a poorly functioning ventricle. He says it is not a major factor in whether he will operate but admits that it is a strong factor in assessing the risk of surgery. His philosophy is that "no matter how poor the ventricle is, if the patient has enough heart muscle to live, but can't tolerate much more damage and what is left is in jeopardy, we'll do it."

If, as is widely accepted, the location, number and size of blockages in the coronary arteries correlate more closely with risk of death from heart disease than do symptoms, *what should be done about patients who have coronary artery disease (as demonstrated by arteriography) but have no symptoms or mild symptoms?* Should they have surgery as a prophylactic measure? Most of these asymptomatic patients had arteriography because they had positive stress tests which suggested the need for further study.

The Cardiology Branch of the National Heart, Lung, and Blood Institute of National Institutes of Health in Bethesda has recently completed a thirty-month follow-up of such patients. Included were 147 who did not have significant lesions of the left main coronary artery and who had ejection fractions greater than 20 percent.

Twenty-eight percent of patients had one-vessel disease; 31 percent had two-vessel disease; and 41 percent had three-vessel disease.

The mortality rate was 1.5 percent per year for single- and double-vessel disease, but 6 percent a year for those with triple-vessel disease.

During the follow-up period, which averaged two years, 40 percent of patients with *triple-vessel disease who did poorly on exercise tests* either died or developed more severe symptoms which required surgery. On the other hand, of the patients with *three-vessel disease who had good exercise capacity,* only 7 percent died and 15 percent developed more serious angina.

The study, headed by Dr. Kenneth M. Kent, *concluded that patients who have no symptoms, or only mild symptoms, and who have single- or double-vessel disease have an excellent prognosis without surgery.* Patients with triple-vessel disease and good exercise capacity on a stress test have an annual mortality rate of 4 percent a year. But patients with triple-vessel disease and poor exercise capacity on a stress test have a poor prognosis. The study concludes that "it appears reasonable to recommend bypass surgery for this subgroup, even in the absence of supporting data derived from a definitive study in which patients were randomized."

Dr. Epstein, of the National Institutes for Health, says that about 70 percent of patients without symptoms have good left ventricular function (ejection fractions of 50 percent or greater) and therefore might be expected to have a good long-term prognosis without surgery. "Studies that indicate a substantially better prognosis for sufferers of two-vessel disease when they receive surgery are based on patients that had severe symptoms," Dr. Epstein says. "But the natural history of patients without such symptoms is quite different."

The NHLBI study points out that the average mortality

rate is only about 2 percent a year in all patients with double-vessel disease, lower than the average mortality rate of surgically treated patients at many institutions.

Another study of fifty-five patients with no symptoms or few symptoms who underwent surgery at the Montreal Heart Institute reinforced the conclusions of the NHLBI study. Of the fifty-five, twenty-one patients had single-vessel disease, thirteen had double-vessel disease, and twenty-seven triple-vessel disease.

No one died in surgery, but two patients had heart attacks following the operation, and three needed second operations to correct persistent bleeding. Soon after the operation, nine of the forty-five grafts had closed. A year later, two patients had all grafts closed, and five years later, another patient, too, had no open grafts. Four patients subsequently died, but only three deaths were related to coronary artery disease. Seven patients had heart attacks later.

The researchers, headed by Dr. Claude M. Grondin, concluded that "it is apparent . . . that patients such as these stand to benefit little from prophylactic [preventive] revascularization. Longevity may be increased, however, in patients who are asymptomatic after heart attack."

And a study conducted by Duke University Medical Center on 1,101 patients who received heart catheterizations between August 1969 and September 1974, reinforcing the findings from the National Institutes of Health, revealed that, *on the average*, coronary artery surgery does not significantly prolong the four-year survival when compared to medical treatment.

The study included patients with blockages of 70 percent or more in at least one coronary artery. Four hundred nine patients received surgery, and 611 were treated medically. However, 21 of the 611 medically treated patients had surgery more than six months after they were catheterized.

At the end of four years, the survival rate of the patients who had operations was 82 percent. It was 78 percent in patients who did not have surgery.

"When groups were compared, it was apparent that what differences there were could be attributed to baseline inequalities, rather than the method of treatment," say the investigators. For example, nonoperated patients were older and had more abnormalities, including more three-vessel disease, more diffuse disease of distal vessels and a higher incidence of poor ventricular function than did the group who received surgery.

The study concludes: "It is probable that for the average patient with coronary artery disease, bypass surgery does not significantly prolong life over a four-year period.

"But one never has to decide how to treat the average patient. What one needs to know is what will happen to a specific patient if treated medically or surgically."

A team at Duke University Medical Center has developed a process, through use of a digital computer, to answer more accurately specific questions about specific patients. It enables physicians to predict what will probably happen to an individual if he or she is treated medically or surgically. It is based on Duke's past experience with surgical and medical patients; a new patient is matched against former patients with similar characteristics.

In the ten years since 1971, when it was developed, Duke's computer data bank has accumulated information on 3,000 patients. The information stored in the computer includes for each patient:

A narrative of present illness;
A checklist of past history;
Results of physical examination;

Laboratory data;
X-ray findings;
Descriptions of coronary vessels;
Test results;
Ventricular function;
Reason for admission;
History of medication or other treatment, including types and dosages;
If surgery were carried out, the procedure and complications.

All patients are followed up at six months, one year and annually thereafter; and additional information about the patient's condition, medication and complications at those times are programmed into the computer.

For new patients, the computer is used as follows.

First, the patient's physician fills in a requisition on which he lists data about his patient. Consider, for example, Jill K., a fifty-six-year-old woman. Jill has stable angina, has three-vessel disease with no obstruction in her left main coronary artery. Her left ventricle is normal.

These are the basic criteria which describe Jill's condition and which are fed into the computer. Her physician would then classify Jill based on myriad characteristics including, among other factors:

· Sex;
· Age;
· Duration of heart disease;
· Whether or not typical angina;
· Progress of chest pain;
· Patient's heart-attack history;
· Hypertension;
· Diabetes;
· Smoking habits;
· Whether treated medically with beta-blockers (an

effective medication in controlling angina—see Chapter 6);

- Ventricular gallop (a heart sound often the first sign of congestive heart failure);
- Peripheral bruit/s (turbulence in an artery usually caused by plaque in a vessel);
- Heart enlargement;
- Abnormalities in the electrocardiogram;
- Positive exercise test;
- Whether the patient had to stop in an early stage on the exercise test;
- Left ventricular end-diastolic pressure;
- Cardiac index (output of the heart corrected for body size);
- Whether ejection fraction is less than 40 percent;
- Three-vessel disease;
- Left ventricular aneurysms (A scarred area of the heart in which a lot of blood can be sequestered. This is present only in some patients who have had heart attacks and, depending on the size of the aneurysm, can compromise left ventricular function.);
- Disease of more than 50 percent of the left main coronary artery.

This information would then be fed into the computer, which would call up the subgroup of patients with characteristics similar to Jill's. The computer would reveal how these patients fared, whether treated surgically or medically. And this information would help Jill and her physician determine her treatment.

Consider John, a forty-three-year-old man, who presented himself at Duke in 1974 with a three-month history of typical angina. His chest pain occurred with exertion and had been infrequent and stable during the ninety-day period.

John was given an exercise test which was negative and during which his heart achieved a maximum heart rate of 180 beats a minute. A subsequent cardiac catheterization showed that his left ventricle was functioning normally, but that John had three-vessel coronary disease. His circumflex artery was totally blocked and there were serious blockages in his left anterior descending and right coronary arteries.

John's *prognostigram* (the name given to the computer analysis) characterized him as having stable chest pain, three-vessel coronary artery disease, no blockage in his left main coronary artery and a normal left ventricle.

The computer called up a sub-group of one hundred seventy-seven patients with these characteristics. All were male. Ninety-two patients had been treated medically and eighty-five had received bypass surgery. The prognostigram showed that there was excellent survival with either medical or surgical treatment.

Because John was not having pain which did not respond to medical management, it was decided to treat him medically.

At this writing, he is doing well with no limitation on his activities and with infrequent episodes of angina.

Another patient, Ben, was forty-three when he was evaluated at Duke in 1975, one month after he had begun to experience angina. Cardiac catheterization showed that Ben, too, had a healthy left ventricle, but there was an almost total occlusion of his left anterior descending coronary artery.

The computer recalled seventy-nine men who were Ben's age, who had had angina less than two years and who had blockages in only one coronary artery (not the left main).

Of these, thirty-four patients had been treated medically and forty-five patients had been treated surgically.

At the end of seven years, there was 96.2 percent mortality rate among those treated medically and a 92.4 percent mortality rate among those treated surgically. Since Ben had not yet been treated adequately with a medical program, he was begun on a medical regimen.

Three years later, he was feeling well and was free of pain.

"The excellent studies on the natural history of patients with coronary artery disease are not always helpful to doctors who want to determine long-term therapy of an individual patient," says Dr. Robert A. Rosati, associate professor of medicine at Duke University Medical Center. "The doctor has no quick way to assess the prognosis of his patient against the experience of similar patients or to know what the effect of treatment will be on the prognosis. Therefore, physicians have had to focus on short-term goals, such as relief of pain. But relief of pain is not closely coupled to survival."

The computer bank gives physicians new information in a form not available in textbooks or journal articles. "Physicians using the data bank can identify in seconds conditions in patients similar to the patient they have and find out what happened to those patients with or without different forms of therapy," Dr. Rosati explains.

Duke University has used its computerized data bank to study relief of pain and survival achieved with medical or surgical treatment. It looked at 781 patients with significant coronary artery disease who were evaluated at Duke's Medical Center between August 1, 1969, and April 20, 1973. Significant disease was defined as 70 percent or greater stenosis (blockage) in any artery. There were 402 patients in the group treated medically and 379 in the surgical group.

Duke's study revealed that:

1. More surgical patients experienced total pain relief. At the end of two years, more than twice as many surgical survivors were pain-free.

2. Surgery does not affect the overall two-year survival. At the end of two years, 83 percent of the medically treated group and 85 percent of the surgically treated group were alive.

3. Patients with three-vessel disease, a localized area of disturbance in ventricular functioning but whose hearts are able to meet the oxygen demands of the body, seem to have a higher two-year survival when treated surgically. These are patients who are theoretically at high risk of heart attack. (More recent experience at Duke indicates that the group of patients with three-vessel disease but which has normal left ventricles and hearts that are able to meet the body's oxygen demands do *not* do better when treated surgically).

4. A low-risk subgroup (patients with one-vessel disease; patients with two-vessel disease and a normal left ventriculogram; and patients with three-vessel disease, a normal ventriculogram and the capacity of the heart to meet the body's oxygen demands) does well with either treatment.

"In the long run, we don't see much of a benefit of surgery in low-risk patients in terms of survival," Dr. Rosati says. He defines low-risk patients as those with an efficiently pumping heart and who do not have left main disease. This low-risk group includes persons with three-vessel disease if their hearts pump efficiently and if they do not have left main disease.

"Once you know such factors as the type of chest pain, the heart size, the response to exercise and the data learned at catheterization, other risk factors, such as hypertension, diabetes, smoking and high cholesterol, don't seem to make much of a difference," says Dr. Rosati. "This is true in the beginning. When we get out past five or ten years, we may find that those other risk factors turn out to be more important."

"The hard part with treating a patient medically," explains Dr. Rosati, "is that you have to be constantly vigilant and constantly reinforcing the patient to take proper care of himself. Surgery is undoubtedly difficult to do and it takes a great deal of training to do it properly; but once it has been done, it is not redone on a week-to-week and month-to-month basis. This is different from medical management.

"Our position is conservative. We have been impressed with how well medically treated patients do."

Emory's Dr. Hurst, however, cautions that delaying surgery in some patients may result in their condition worsening to the point where they are no longer candidates for surgery. He cites his experience with twenty-four patients with unstable angina, all with double- or triple-vessel disease. All had surgery. At the end of a two-year follow-up, all were alive.

Dr. Hurst compares this with results reported by Drs. C. Richard Conti and G. D. Plotnick from the Johns Hopkins Hospital and the University of Florida at Gainesville, who separated patients with unstable angina into two groups. Group I included patients who were considered suitable for surgery but did not have it. Group II consisted of patients who were inoperable. At the end of the first year, the mortality rate in Group I was 9.5 percent. There were no additional deaths in the next three years.

"I find it difficult and believe it to be unwise to delay surgery," says Dr. Hurst, "when it is clear that many patients will die or become inoperable if one just waits and hopes that all goes well."

Duke investigators emphasize that coronary artery disease is a chronic condition. Patients who are low-risk today may be at considerably greater risk a year or two later. Their arteries may become more clogged. Their left ventricles may function less efficiently. Other risk factors, such as hypertension or high cholesterol, may have taken their toll.

Whatever the decisions are that are made by patients and their doctors at a given time, they must be re-evaluated from time to time, based on the patient's symptoms and the results of new testing.

5 WHAT IS THE OPERATION LIKE, AND WHAT ARE THE RISKS?

Vincent D., a fifty-eight-year-old man with triple-vessel coronary artery disease, sits in his bed at Philadelphia's Lankenau Hospital, talking cheerfully about the heart-bypass operation he is scheduled to have the next morning.

Vincent has been in pain since 1972. He has had four heart catheterizations, has not been able to work and has been in and out of fifteen hospitals. "I was taking fifty pills a day," he says. "Everybody kept telling me I had coronary artery disease, but that I was not a candidate for the operation. My blockages were not big enough—they were only about 40 or 50 percent. But now they say I am a candidate.

"Do you want to know how I feel? I'm scared, really scared. But I'd have been more scared if they told me they couldn't do anything for me. I was going off my rocker with the pain."

Later that afternoon, a critical-care specialist visited Vincent to tell him what he could expect the next day. The specialist has already given Vincent and his family an orientation to surgery. She holds classes during which she describes to patients and their relatives what will be happening to them. She tries to relieve their anxiety. "We find that when they are less anxious, less scared, they can be more cooperative because they know what we are doing and why we are doing it," she says.

The specialist describes the procedure to Vincent in meticulous detail. "Someone will come in tonight to shave your body," she tells him. "That's to keep the danger of infection down and to keep it from hurting too much when we have to take the bandages off.

"At five-thirty in the morning, you will get a needle and a pill while you are in your room, to make you feel drowsy. At six-thirty you will come to the operating room. Don't be frightened by the equipment you will see there. It looks a little like a scene out of *Star Wars*, but it is all supposed to be there. It doesn't mean anything is wrong.

"I'll meet you in the operating room. You'll see a lot of me while you're here," she tells him.

The next morning, Vincent is wheeled to surgery. He is unusually alert. "Hope you had a good night's sleep," he tells his surgeon, Dr. Horace MacVaugh.

Vincent is moved to the operating table where he lies flat on his back, his arms spread to the sides. The anesthesiologist and his team are ready. The circulating nurse is counting the instruments needed for the operation. The heart-lung machine that will oxygenate and circulate Vincent's blood during the surgery is wheeled in.

The anesthesiologist explains what will happen. "We will be putting an oxygen line in your nose. Then you'll get an IV [intravenous] needle in your arm. We'll be putting a catheter into the radial artery in your wrist so we can monitor your arterial blood pressure directly. I'm going to put another catheter into the jugular vein in your neck. It will go into the right side of your heart to monitor pressure and blood gases. You'll feel a little stick, and it may burn slightly. But it shouldn't feel too bad."

Vincent is still awake when the catheter is inserted, but

soon afterward the anesthesiologist tells him, "You're going to go to sleep now. I'll see you in the special-care unit in about four hours. Everything is fine, and it's going to stay that way. Have a good sleep."

Now, with Vincent asleep on the table, the anesthesiologist slips an endotracheal tube through Vincent's vocal chords and into the trachea to permit him to breathe until the heart-lung machine takes over. The tube will not be taken out until later that day or the next morning, when it is certain that Vincent can breathe on his own.

Now Vincent is ready to be "painted." The surgical assistant swabs his whole body with an antiseptic solution the color of rusty water. "This decreases the number of bacteria on his body," she says. "They'll give him a bath in the intensive-care unit and wipe all of this stuff off." Plastic sheeting is placed over Vincent's body to further shield him, and he is draped in green surgical fabric so that only the chest area to be worked on and his legs are exposed.

During the next four hours, surgical assistants will remove the saphenous veins from Vincent's legs, and Dr. MacVaugh will delicately stitch them to the diseased vessels, bypassing Vincent's obstructions and permitting blood to flow freely to his heart. During this time, Vincent will be monitored constantly for pressure, samples of his blood will be checked by the laboratory every few minutes (and the results called in to the operating room) and his urine output will be measured frequently.

Vincent will not be breathing on his own but will be connected to a heart-lung machine that will take over his breathing and blood circulation during the surgery. (It is the heart-lung machine, as discussed earlier, that makes this kind of surgery possible.) The machine will take all the venous blood which would normally return to Vincent's heart, will oxygenate it, remove the carbon dioxide and return it to the arterial side of his circulation, through sets of tubing, at the appropriate pressure and rate of flow to support his vital functions. A spinning roller pump pushes blood through the tubing at a rate of five or six quarts a minute.

All of this is done at a preselected temperature—usually between 24 and 32 degrees centigrade—which will cool his body. "We want to cool the body down because a cold body demands less oxygen," explains Dr. MacVaugh. "The temperature we select depends partially on the anticipated duration of the operation."

Just before Vincent is connected to the heart-lung machine, the anesthesiologist gives him a big dose of heparin, an anticoagulant that will keep his blood from clotting during surgery.

By 9:30 A.M. the veins from his leg have been removed and put into a saline solution to keep until Dr. MacVaugh is ready for them.

A vertical incision is made in the center of Vincent's chest, his breastbone is sawed in half and the skin clamped back to reveal the mustard-color gelatinous mass that is the heart. Actually, the heart is usually pinkish in color, but in Vincent's case the accumulation of fat makes it appear yellowish.

Dr. MacVaugh pours an ice-cold saline solution over the heart, which is strong and muscular, to cool it even more than the rest of the body. Then he gently lifts the heart so he can wrap a cardiac support (jokingly referred to by the surgical team as a "cardiac jockstrap") around it. It is important to keep the heart still while the surgeons work.

The scrub nurse hands Dr. MacVaugh a saphenous vein, a 12-inch-long segment which looks as though it could slip through a straw. The vein must be just the right length, not long enough to kink or short enough to be taut. After Dr. MacVaugh has tested it to be sure it is open, he sutures one end of it to a tiny opening he has cut in the artery branch, just below the obstruction. Dr. MacVaugh wears three-and-a-half-power magnifying telescopic lenses; the stitching is tedious, meticulous and requires deft fingering. The process is repeated three times, one for each of the bypasses. In Vincent's case, there are bypasses to the right coronary artery, the circumflex artery and the left anterior descending artery.

Then the other end of each vein is attached to a small hole which Dr. MacVaugh has punched in the aorta, the huge vessel which carries blood out of the heart and distributes it through the body.

While Dr. MacVaugh is attaching the vein to the aorta, he gives instructions to begin rewarming Vincent's body. The operator of the heart-lung machine achieves this by raising the temperature of the water in the machine's heat exchanger.

Now four slim pacemaker wires are attached directly to Vincent's heart. They are brought out through his chest wall, just below his incision. An external pacemaker, about the size of a small portable radio, is connected to them. Its purpose is to efficiently handle any problems of arrhythmia or drop in heart rate that might occur. "You hope he will come right off bypass [the heart-lung machine] with no trouble, but this is a safeguard," Dr. MacVaugh explains. Vincent will wear the pacemaker until he leaves the hospital, at which time the pacemaker wires can be easily withdrawn.

Dr. MacVaugh checks to be certain his patient's condition is stable. "OK, let's go off bypass," he says. The machine operator slows and finally stops the heart-lung machine, while the anesthesiologist begins to ventilate Vincent's lungs. As he does this, Vincent's heart swells to its full size and begins to take over its normal pumping function.

Now Dr. MacVaugh checks Vincent's vital signs and

inspects his grafts to be certain there are no kinks or leaks. He is satisfied and gives instructions to disconnect the heart-lung machine.

At the same time, the anesthesiologist administers protamine to neutralize the effect of the heparin given earlier. Now Vincent's blood will begin to clot again.

Dr. MacVaugh makes two short skin incisions through which he inserts plastic chest tubes to drain blood and serum that normally accumulate after major surgery.

The final steps are pulling the breastbone together with stainless-steel wires that remain in place permanently (generally they cause no discomfort to the patient) and suturing the incision.

The operation is over. Vincent has been on the table for just under five hours.

He is ready to be moved to the intensive-care unit, where he will remain for twenty-four hours. This is a crucial time, and the anesthesiologist connects him to a battery-powered monitor for the trip. The monitor will record electrocardiographic readings and blood-pressure tracings during the transfer.

The intensive-care unit has no day or night. Specially trained nurses hover over the patients every moment. Monitors record vital signs. Buzzers ring. Nurses have learned to recognize early signs and symptoms in a patient that call for prompt treatment. In many cardiac-care units, nurses have been authorized by physicians to perform vital procedures to correct irregularities of the heartbeat or other complications that may arise.

When Vincent reached the cardiac-care unit, he was still asleep. His family was told that it would be several hours before he would be awake and able to see them. Tubes would probably remain in his nose and throat during that time and up to twenty-four hours, depending on how well he seemed able to breathe on his own.

A nurse in the cardiac-care unit taped electrodes to

Vincent's chest and legs. These were to help pick up signals from the heart and relay them to the heart monitor that is carefully watched by the nurses at his bed and in the nursing station. Occasionally, an electrode loosens, and the monitor will sound an alarm. Vincent had been told in advance not to be frightened if this occurred. The signal would not mean that there was any irregularity in his heart action.

Continuous checks of Vincent's breathing, blood pressure, temperature, pulse and skin color were taken. Nurses tried to talk to him and, the moment he stirred, asked him how he felt.

Vincent smiled faintly and tugged at the tube in his throat. The nurses knew what he meant. The tube in the throat is often the most uncomfortable part of the procedure. Fortunately, most patients can have it removed shortly after surgery.

In Vincent's case, the tube was removed twelve hours after he left the operating room. From that time on, he was encouraged to breathe deeply and cough, to clear fluid from his lungs. The next day, Vincent was removed from the intensive-care unit and taken to a private room. He was able to leave his bed to use the bathroom, walking slowly and with the support of a nurse.

"I was surprised how quickly I was able to walk around and feel fairly comfortable," Vincent says. "I had some pain, especially in the area where the incision was, and my legs bothered me a little where they had cut, but I improved rapidly."

In ten days, Vincent left the hospital. The thing he remembers most about his operation is the "beautiful" nurses in the intensive-care unit. "I can't tell you how much difference they make," he says. "They are there all the time, and they know just what to do for you."

Vincent still has some discomfort from his incision, but

otherwise he is free of the crippling angina pain he suffered for so many years.

"Today [fifteen days after surgery], I took a walk outside for the first time," Vincent says. "Down to the mailbox to mail some letters. In the letters I told people how I feel. I told them I feel as though I were reborn. My new birthday is June 1 [the day of his surgery]. I'm starting over, and I have a whole new life."

Because Vincent and thousands like him come through surgery without a mishap, and because so much bypass surgery is performed, there is sometimes a tendency to underestimate the seriousness of a heart-bypass operation. It is not a procedure to be taken lightly, nor is it without risk.

It is an operation where the skill of the surgical team is critical; in fact, mortality rates vary widely, and the outcome of the operation may well depend on who does it and where it is done. "This is the most highly technical of any cardiac surgery, and I've been watching for thirty years," says cardiologist Dr. George G. Rowe at the University of Wisconsin. "All you have to do is get one stitch out of place. . . . If you don't do it right, it won't do."

Major medical centers where cardiac surgery is performed routinely by a skilled surgical team—centers such as Cleveland Clinic, Texas Heart Institute, Deborah Heart and Lung Center, Baylor College of Medicine, University of Wisconsin, University of Alabama—enjoy lower mortality rates than hospitals where heart-bypass surgery is a less frequent occurrence. And the number of operations performed by a surgeon correlates closely with the success of the operation. Dr. Denton Cooley, one of the country's leading heart surgeons, and his team do more than 2,800 bypass operations every year.

Dr. Cooley is tall, elegant—the ultimate gentleman—and he takes in his stride the crushing pressure of his work, his fame and his incredibly jammed schedule. On a typical day, he might supervise thirty operations and participate directly in fifteen of those. When surgery is over, he reports to each patient's family, giving them the final word (even though they have received hourly reports on the patient's progress).

Like other surgical teams whose specialty is open-heart surgery, Dr. Cooley's operating-room staff functions with assembly-line precision. There is no time to waste, no margin for error. In fact, the section in which his operating rooms are located is often called "the heart-surgery factory." His patients worship him, and he assures them when he makes his rounds, "Don't worry. We'll take good care of you. We'll make you well."

Nonetheless, even in the deft hands of Dr. Denton Cooley, Dr. Floyd Loop, Dr. Gerald Lemole, Dr. Dudley Johnson, Dr. N. T. Kouchoukos, Dr. John Kirklin and others of similar skill and reputation, there are risks of which patients should be aware.

"Most people, except for engineers and drug salesmen, are timid about confronting their doctors," says Milwaukee's Dr. Johnson. "Ask them, 'What are the risks? What are my chances? How many such operations have you done? What is your mortality rate? What percentage of your grafts stay open?' "

Some physicians, for instance, are better able to work with smaller vessels than others; some are more willing than others to operate on patients who do not have efficiently functioning left ventricles. In fact, it is not uncommon for a patient to be refused surgery at one hospital and accepted at another. The Cleveland Clinic, the University of Wisconsin, the Texas Heart Institute of St. Luke's Episcopal Hospital and other large centers see many patients who have been rejected by other hospitals.

Charles is a case in point. Five years ago, he had a

double-bypass operation at a Philadelphia hospital. For the first three years following his surgery, his angina was dramatically relieved. But in the beginning of the fourth year, he began to experience pain again. It was mild at first but increased in intensity and eventually became more severe than the pain which had sent him to surgery in the first place.

Medication gave him no relief, and his cardiologist scheduled him for another coronary catheterization. It revealed that one of his original bypasses had become blocked and that his right coronary artery, which was not significantly occluded at the time of the earlier surgery, was also 90 percent blocked. In addition, he had diffuse disease, meaning that many of his distal branch arteries were clogged. Surgeons at his original hospital told him that a re-operation would be too risky for him and that his disease was too widespread for them to tackle.

Charles was sent back to his cardiologist for medical treatment. However, his pain intensified until finally he was confined to bed, convinced that the doctors had sent him home to die.

A friend suggested that he see another doctor in Washington, D.C., where Charles and his family had moved. Another catheterization was performed, and the results were compared with the earlier studies.

Charles was told that because he had a poorly functioning left ventricle (ejection fraction of 25 percent) and diffuse disease, he would be a riskier candidate for surgery than he was at the time of his earlier operation. But the surgeon was confident that he would survive the operation successfully.

"I had no choice," Charles says. "I was incapacitated." The surgery was performed in August 1980. Charles made an excellent recovery, is back at work and is free of pain. "I've always been a believer in second opinions," he says. "But with heart surgery, it isn't even an option. It is a must."

Patients who are considering heart-bypass surgery are concerned about the risks of the operation. And there is a tendency for a person who has been told he needs, for instance, a triple bypass to compare himself with a friend or relative who has also had a triple bypass. If the friend had little trouble, he feels reassured, hopeful that he will have the same experience. On the other hand, if the friend developed complications, he is fearful that he, too, faces the same danger.

It is not so. The risks involved in heart surgery depend largely on characteristics of the specific patient before he or she ever enters the operating room, factors such as age, sex, location of the blockages, health of the heart muscle, presence or absence of diabetes, heart failure, heart-valve problems, history of heart attack or other heart disease.

Risks are greater for older patients because their tissue is more brittle; risks are greater for women than men, probably because their arteries are thinner and smaller (not as easy to bypass). Those with poorly functioning left ventricles are at greater risk because their heart muscle is damaged. And disease of the left main coronary artery, because of its critical location and function, imposes greater surgical risk than blockages located elsewhere. The general health of the person, of course, also counts heavily.

Of these preoperative risk factors, it is felt that the number and location of the blockages and the condition of the left ventricle may indeed be the most significant.

A study conducted in Seattle which looked at risk factors in 121 bypass patients found that, of the patients who did not survive surgery, the performance of the left ventricle was substantially abnormal. There was a tenfold increase in mortality in patients whose ejection fraction (which measures the function of the left ventricle) was less than 33 percent. Interestingly, patients with only moderately impaired ventricles did not seem to have a higher surgical mortality.

Another study from Vanderbilt University Medical School in Nashville found that a "bad" left ventricle, left main disease, a recent heart attack and aortic or mitral valve disease are highly predictive of increased surgical risk. Other risk factors, such as age, sex, history of past heart attack or severity of angina, were found to be less significant to *immediate* survival.

"There is no question that the operative risk is higher for persons whose left ventricle is not functioning efficiently," says Dr. Gerald Lemole. If the damage is moderate, Dr. René Favaloro, one of the originators of bypass surgery, feels it can be done with a mortality rate of about 1 or 2 percent. Where the damage is serious, the mortality is higher.

Consider, for instance, Judith L. and Leonard T. Both have blockages of 75 percent in the right coronary artery, 70 percent in the left anterior descending artery and 80 percent in the circumflex. Both will require triple bypass operations, but their operative risk is starkly different.

Judith is sixty, female, has congestive heart failure and has had one heart attack. Her ejection fraction is 30, which means that her heart muscle is not operating as efficiently as it should. All of these characteristics increase her risk.

Leonard, on the other hand, is male, fifty, has a healthy heart muscle with an ejection fraction of 75 and no other heart problems. His risk, of course, is considerably lower.

Chances are that both Judith and Leonard will survive the operation without problems. New techniques and more sophisticated surgical procedures have contributed to an operative risk which is surprisingly low when one considers the gravity of the operation.

Many patients complain that while their doctors admitted to them that bypass surgery entails some risk, they did not explain why or give them enough knowledge to weigh the risks against the benefits. But results of a recent large-scale study, perhaps the most definitive on preoperative risk, may help.

Fifteen centers participated in the Collaborative Study in Coronary Artery Surgery (CASS). Its goal was to understand the characteristics in a patient that predict operative mortality. Participating centers included the University of Alabama, Albany Medical College, Loma Linda University, Boston University, Marshfield Clinical Foundation for Medical Research and Education, Massachusetts General Hospital, Mayo Clinic and Mayo Foundation, Miami Heart Institute, Montreal Heart Institute, New York University, St. Louis University, St. Luke's Hospital Center, Stanford University, Medical College of Wisconsin and Yale University. The University of Washington was the coordinating center, and the study was carried out under the auspices of the National Heart, Lung, and Blood Institute.

In order of importance, the predictors were:

- Age. Persons under sixty had a mortality rate of 1.4 percent, while those older than sixty had a mortality rate of 4.2 percent.
- Presence of blockage in the left main coronary artery of more than 90 percent which makes surgery more complex.
- Left ventricular dysfunction. It has long been known, and the CASS study confirms, that this characteristic is associated with increased operative mortality.

Other factors that predict risk during or soon after surgery are: sex, with females being at greater risk; the presence of severe and/or unstable angina; signs of heart failure; the number of arteries with more than 70 percent blockages; and the type of surgery—whether it was elective, urgent or an emergency; whether there were other procedures necessary in addition to bypass (for instance, mitral valve replacement); and the number of arteries bypassed.

In 4,303 patients under sixty who had bypass surgery alone, the operative mortality was 1.4 percent, and the most important characteristics were sex and whether or not patients had congestive heart failure. But in 1,873 patients older than sixty where the mortality was 4.2 percent, left main disease (with more than 90 percent blockages) and unstable angina were the most important predictors.

When patients were separated into three groups and evaluated on the basis of their need for surgery—elective, urgent or emergency—the operative mortality was at least twice as high for women in all categories.

Between August 1975 and December 31, 1978, the mortality rate was 2.1 percent in 1975 and 1976; 2.3 percent in 1977; and 2.6 percent in 1978; no statistically significant difference during that period.

Interestingly, in contrast to other studies, the number of vessels bypassed (except when the left main artery was involved) did not seem to have significant bearing on operative mortality.

Despite the increased risks to people who are older, thousands of men and women in their late sixties and seventies come through bypass surgery remarkably well. Julia W. is such a woman. No one believed that Julia was seventy-four. Her face was smooth and unlined, framed by still-brown hair that fell softly to her shoulders. She played tennis, rode a bicycle four miles every day and swam at the neighborhood community center. She still worked as a receptionist in a physician's office three mornings a week and reassured patients with her easy conversation, confident attitude and bright smile.

Julia had been having angina which has increased in intensity for the past two years. But as long as she was able to continue her active life-style, she did not consider surgery. She knew that her age and sex put her at higher risk.

But sixteen months ago, Julia experienced pain that was more severe, so stunning, in fact, that she had to be hospitalized so that her condition could be brought under control. Her physician urged that she have a catheterization, which showed an 85 percent blockage in her left main coronary artery. Now there was an additional and critical risk factor if she chose to have surgery. But her physician felt that she was at greater risk if she did not.

Julia went to the hairdresser the day before she entered the hospital. She had a manicure, pedicure, facial and had her hair cut a little shorter ("so it wouldn't get all matted down and hard to take care of while I was in the hospital"). She bought a few new nightgowns with buttons down the front so that doctors could get to her incision when they had to examine her. "I didn't want to wear those hospital gowns. They are so depressing," she said.

She asked a longtime friend to take care of her mail and left with her a sealed envelope with instructions to follow in case of her death.

"I was much more frightened than I would admit," Julia remembers. "I knew I wasn't a prime candidate for this operation, and I wasn't sure I'd ever come out of it. But I was determined to put on a happy face, and if I went [died], I was going to go in style and dignity."

Julia was able to keep her happy face. There were no complications during her surgery. Her main problem, she says, was to keep coughing after the operation. "The nurses kept annoying me to cough, and it was so painful to do it. But I didn't get pneumonia or anything, so I know they knew what they were doing."

Today, Julia's schedule is as jammed as it was before she had the operation. Her doctors credit her recovery to a positive mental attitude and excellent physical health, except for her heart problems.

"I had to have the operation," Julia says. "I enjoy living too much to give up on myself without a struggle."

Julia was fortunate to have a strong heart muscle, but the presence of left main disease put her at greater risk of operative mishap. Most patients with this condition also have widespread coronary artery disease, and almost two-thirds of them have serious obstructions of their right coronary artery. Julia did not.

At the Cleveland Clinic, Dr. Floyd Loop says that the operative mortality for patients with left main disease has dropped from 4 percent in earlier years to 1.2 percent in 1979. And Dr. Michael DeBakey, chancellor of the Baylor College of Medicine in Houston, says that his institution does not consider age per se as a risk factor. The oldest patient on whom Dr. DeBakey and his team operated was eighty-seven. The patient is now ninety-two and doing well.

Julia was fortunate also not to have suffered from a recent heart attack before her surgery. A report on 1,700 patients from the Texas Heart Institute shows a 38 percent mortality when the patient has had a heart attack eight to thirty days before the operation, and a 5.8 percent mortality when the heart attack was thirty-one to sixty days old. It is generally preferable for surgery to be postponed, if possible, for approximately three months after heart attack.

Although Julia's operation involved only one bypass, disease of the left main coronary artery is equivalent to multiple-vessel disease and carried the biggest surgical risk of all.

Studies produce conflicting results about the relationship between number of bypasses to mortality. For instance, Emory University's study of more than 3,000 men and women operated on between July 1973 and December 1979 indicates that the death rate was 2 out of 637 patients with single-vessel disease; 8 deaths of 981 patients for double-vessel disease; and 18 deaths of 1,046 patients with triple-vessel disease. Left main disease had a mortality rate of 12 patients out of 470. The in-hospital death rate was higher for women than for men in the categories of single- and triple-vessel disease.

On the other hand, an analysis of what it is that affects hospital mortality by Dr. N. T. Kouchoukos and his associates at the University of Alabama found that, despite the increase in the number of grafts per patient from 1970 to 1977, the mortality rate declined, and there was no difference in death rate for those who received two or three grafts, compared with those who received four to seven grafts.

Operative mortality rates (during the operation) and perioperative mortality rates (within thirty days after surgery) vary widely, depending on who is doing the surgery and where it is being done. Dr. George Crile, for twelve years chairman of the Cleveland Clinic's department of surgery, says, "Small hospitals which do only a few bypass operations a year may have ten times the mortality rate of medical centers where surgeons have a great deal of experience." But no matter where the surgery is performed or how skilled the operating team is, complications can occur during or soon after surgery. And there are delayed risks that may not be experienced until months or years later.

Some of the dangers are directly related to the patient's

own risk factors. Others are unexpected, and there is no way to predict who will be affected.

Among the variety of mishaps that can be induced by coronary bypass surgery are:

A Heart Attack

This can occur sometimes because of complications relating to anesthesia; a shift in blood pressure when anesthesia is given can occasionally create an imbalance between supply and demand of oxygen that precipitates a heart attack.

A heart attack is more likely to happen if a person is connected too long to the heart-lung machine. "The quicker we do the procedure and get new blood into the heart, the better," explains Deborah's Dr. Gerald Lemole. "While the heart is on bypass, it gets no blood." Dr. Lemole estimated that the average patient will spend forty-five minutes to an hour hooked up to the machine.

And heart attacks are more frequent in patients with left main disease, those with poor left ventricles and those with widespread disease in the distal vessels of the heart. "People with bad left ventricles have little or no reserve," explains Dr. Lemole. "For a couple of days after surgery, the heart has to work a little harder, and these patients are often already at their limit. They can't recruit any more heart muscle to help them."

For the same reason, patients with damaged heart muscle have no margin for tolerating even the slightest problem that could occur during surgery, and they may suffer a heart attack.

Sometimes a patient may have already suffered an undetected heart attack just before surgery. These men and women are, of course, less able to withstand the strain of surgery superimposed over the myocardial infarction they are experiencing.

Some heart attacks are fatal; of those that are not, some are easily detectable through electrocardiogram readings and measures of blood enzymes. Still other patients suffer heart attacks during surgery and are not even aware of it.

Several studies report that the incidence of such heart attacks has occurred in from 1.3 percent to forty percent of patients in surgery. Kouchoukos and his colleagues at the University of Alabama report that 5 percent of patients at their institution had suffered a heart attack.

Many patients can tolerate a surgically induced heart attack rather well. In fact, it has been said that a heart attack during surgery may even explain the relief of pain that generally follows the operation . . . a dead heart muscle (the result of a heart attack) is insensitive to pain.

Mike P., forty-nine, is a tough-looking factory hand who worked hard and kept to himself. Unlike his coworkers, he went home after work, did not socialize with them and brown-bagged his lunch, which he ate every day while reading philosophy books in the company cafeteria. Each year, Mike would breeze through the company physical. His blood pressure was low-normal. His electrocardiogram was negative. And he had no physical complaints. But one day while at work, he experienced a pressing pain in his chest that vanished in a few minutes. He was taken to the infirmary and given an electrocardiogram, which revealed nothing. When the same kind of incident recurred the following week and the week after, Mike went to his family physician, who diagnosed his problem as angina. However, medication did not help him, and he agreed to have a heart catheterization.

"We couldn't believe there was something wrong with Mike's heart," quipped a coworker. "We never thought he had a heart to go bad."

Mike's heart was indeed "bad." He had three blocked arteries and was advised to have surgery.

"I hardly remember the operation," he says. "I just recall waking up in the intensive-care room with all these monitors and nurses. And I thought it was funny that I stayed in that place five days, when everyone else seemed to move out faster. But I never asked why. And no one ever told me that anything had gone wrong during the operation."

Three months later, before returning to work, Mike had another physical examination by the company doctor. He was stunned when the physician told him that his electrocardiogram showed that he had had a heart attack.

"Then I pieced it together," Mike said. "That was why I was in intensive care so long. I called my surgeon right away and demanded to know. I told him I wanted to see my records. That's when he said that there was some suspicion that I may have had an attack in the operating room, but they couldn't know for sure.

"Well, I'm sure about two things . . . that I had an attack during the surgery, and that they would have never told me about it if I hadn't pressed them."

Does it matter that Mike may have had a heart attack on the operating table as long as he is well now? A study of patients at the University of Alabama reveals that it does. When 1,180 patients, operated on between 1970 and 1975, were followed up for five years, it was found that a heart attack suffered during surgery has far-reaching implications for the future.

Of this group, 799 did not have heart attacks during surgery, as verified by a study of their enzyme levels (enzyme levels are elevated when a heart attack has taken place) and their electrocardiograms, which showed no significant changes. Sixty-eight patients (6 percent) showed both elevated enzyme levels and significant changes on electrocardiograms, which indicated that a heart attack had occurred. Another group of patients—323—was classified as "suspect." Their enzymes were elevated, but their electrocardiograms did not reveal any changes.

As in the case of other studies, the rate of heart attack dropped as the study progressed. It was 13 percent in the earlier years and was reduced to 3 or 3.5 percent in 1974 and 1975. Patients who had the surgery in 1976 and 1977 continued to have heart attacks at the rate of 3.5 percent.

The implications of such surgical heart attacks were dramatic. Thirty-two percent of patients who had an attack during surgery (during 1970–1972) had a heart attack within the next five years; but only 10 percent of those who did not have a heart attack or were in the "suspect" group had one during the same five-year period.

Even during the next three years, when the rate of late heart attack (more than thirty days after surgery) was lower in all three groups, there was still a higher incidence of heart attacks within five years if the person had had one during the operation.

The survival rate, too, correlated with the incidence of heart attack during surgery. For all five years (1970–1975), patients with positive evidence of heart attack had more deaths, patients with suspected heart attacks had fewer deaths and those without heart attacks had the fewest.

Few factors seemed helpful in predicting which patients would have heart attacks during surgery, with the exception of a history of smoking and use of antilipid medications.

Other studies also point out the ominous link between heart attacks during surgery and later prognosis. They suggest that angiograms taken after surgery reveal new blockages, decreased wall motion of the heart (indicating damage) or decline in ejection fraction when a heart attack had been experienced during the operation.

An article published in the *American Heart Journal* reported that typical changes of perioperative myocardial infarction (heart attack within thirty days after surgery) were visible in 40 percent of electrocardiograms taken postoperatively. The patients with this evidence had the highest incidence of death, although there was no difference from patients who survived in the degree of angina, congestive heart failure or history of heart attack prior to surgery.

Argentina's Dr. Favaloro comments that the incidence of postoperative myocardial infarction depends mainly upon the operative technique and the selection of patients. Ideal patients—those with obstruction in the front segment of their arteries, who have good distal vessels and normal left ventricular function—run a low risk of operative or postoperative mortality. But patients with a history of heart attack, widespread disease and abnormal left ventricles run a greater risk of heart attack. They require more time on a heart-lung machine during surgery, which elevates their risk. The incidence of postoperative heart attack in this group of patients has been six percent, in Dr. Favaloro's experience.

What about the rare instance of a heart that cannot be weaned from the heart-lung machine? Replacement of the patient's heart by an artificial one or even a real one may be considered in the future.

Following a triple bypass operation at the Texas Heart Institute in the summer of 1981, the heart of a thirty-six-year-old man would not resume beating. His surgical team, headed by Dr. Denton Cooley, replaced the heart with a plastic pump which remained in place for fifty-four hours until it was replaced with the heart of a twenty-nine-year-old Tennessee laborer who had suffered brain death while undergoing repair of a broken jaw. The new heart started to beat right away and the patient was able to respond to verbal commands such as, "squeeze my hand" or "move your arm."

However, after a week, he died of kidney failure, lung problems and infection. Dr. Cooley said, "Needless to say, it is a disappointment. Nevertheless we can point to the experience to demonstrate that human life can be sustained with a mechanical heart. In this case, we were only able to prolong this man's life for several days. Hopefully, in the future, we can ensure a longer survival."

Brain and Nerve Injury

In the best-selling book *Heartsounds,* Martha Weinman Lear describes her husband's neurologic problems suffered after heart-bypass surgery. His memory failed, and he grew increasingly perturbed with himself because he could not function with his customary efficiency and vigor. Yet Ms. Lear and her physician husband could not get a doctor to talk freely with them about the neurological complications that are sometimes the legacy of heart surgery.

Indeed, there is little information in medical journals about the subject. One such paper was presented at the 1980 meetings of the American Heart Association. It was based on a study by Dr. A. C. Breuer and a team of physicians at the Cleveland Clinic of 421 consecutive patients undergoing bypass surgery to assess the frequency, nature and mechanism of neurological damage. All patients were examined by a neurologist before and once or twice following surgery, beginning on the fourth day after the operation. Approximately 451 characteristics were assessed in each patient that might give clues as to risk. The group included 361 men and 60 women, ranging in age from 36 to 78. For most of the patients—379—it was their first bypass operation. Forty-two patients were having heart surgery for the second time. Twelve percent of patients had single-vessel disease, 32 percent two-vessel disease and 56 percent had three-vessel disease.

The study found that:

- The frequency of damage to the central nervous system (stroke), which would significantly affect a person's functioning, was low, about 2 percent.
- The most common neurological complication was a transient state of confusion, which resolved itself, in most cases, by the time of discharge. This is the kind of thing that might manifest itself by disorientation and transient difficulty with memory.

Fifty-five patients developed new nervous-system problems that were not related to the brain or spinal cord. There were transient forms of injuries to the nerves in the arms and legs.

Patients experiencing such problems had symptoms of weakness or tingling of the hand, arm or shoulder; hoarseness of the voice; facial weakness; drooping of an eyelid; or weakness in a foot. Some patients complained of numbness of their fourth and fifth fingers and weakness and clumsiness of their hand. All of these patients tended to improve, but some had residual weakness and numbness of the hand. The vast majority recovered without significant disability.

These different types of neurologic injuries were not related to the age or sex of the patient, to the presence of diabetes or to the amount of time spent on the heart-lung machine during surgery. "From the massive amount of information analyzed, it was not possible to predict which patient would develop these kinds of problems," says Dr. Breuer. "Further studies are in progress to probe more deeply into this question."

Melvin M., fifty-six, remembers that the major problem he experienced when he returned from the hospital after a triple-bypass operation was extreme clumsiness in his right hand. He was unable to hold a pen without shaking, and he often had trouble getting a fork or spoon to his mouth without dropping the food that was on it. "It was a terrible, helpless, frustrating feeling," Melvin says. "It makes you feel as though you are losing control, and it affects your image of yourself. For a few months, I didn't want to go out in public. I was too embarrassed. But my doctors kept telling me that it would go away. And they were right. After six or seven months, my hand began to get stronger. And now [three years later] I have no problem at all."

"Neurological complications are rare—about one percent in my experience," says Deborah Hospital's Dr. Gerald Lemole. "The most common is a stroke which can show itself in a paralysis of one side, not being able to talk, blindness—depending on which area of the brain was affected."

The most common cause is probably an air bubble, a bit of calcium or a small clot that breaks off and escapes to the brain. Older people who have more widespread arteriosclerosis, which may affect the brain, are more susceptible. So are persons with lesions in their carotid arteries (the pulsating arteries on either side of the neck).

In the early days of the surgery, the mental confusion and forgetfulness that many patients exhibited after the operation were often attributed to a small stroke. However, it is now felt that the emotional stress of so serious an operation and the time lag suffered by patients in intensive-care units may be more responsible.

"You have to remember that a person wakes up in an intensive-care unit—a place that has no windows, where it is always daylight, where there is always activity," says Dr. Lemole. "He [or she] has just been through a gigantic operation and now feels as though he is in a war zone. It is not so unusual to be confused, to wonder what day it is or what time it is."

Minor strokes also used to be blamed on microparticles that might escape from the heart-lung machine. But today, improved equipment virtually eliminates that possibility.

Postoperative Bleeding

This complication has been called the second most common problem that can arise from heart-bypass surgery. Actually, many surgeons say that it is not very common in bypass patients but is higher in persons who undergo heart-valve surgery, because there is more cutting necessary. Almost no one dies from postoperative bleeding, but the condition can be frightening, annoying and require a longer stay in the hospital.

Richard L., sixty-seven, was such a patient. After a double-bypass operation with no complications, he began to bleed while in the intensive-care unit. "I didn't know anything about what complications there could be or how serious they could be when I went into the hospital," says Richard, "so I was scared to death when I knew I was bleeding. I thought I was dying. The nurses kept reassuring me I was going to be OK, but I didn't believe them. They told me they were calling the doctor, but I knew they had gone to call the priest. I was so sure that when the doctor came, I asked him, 'What are you doing here?' "

Richard had to stay in the hospital for an extra week

because of the bleeding, but he recovered well and it did not affect him later.

Wound Infection

Bypass surgery carries a small risk of wound infection (infection at the site of the incision); however, the risk is low and is considerably less than with many other operations, including abdominal surgery or certain kinds of plastic surgery. When an infection does occur, it is important that it be drained promptly to avoid spreading into the bloodstream, which can result in death.

Extent of Revascularization

When bypass surgery originated in the late 1960s, it was felt that the risk of mortality increased with the number of bypass grafts inserted. It was expected that the use of more bypasses indicated the presence of more serious disease in the coronary arteries, and there were more grafts with which something could go wrong. Indeed, patients who were told they needed four or five bypasses were terrified about the implications of this kind of surgery for their prognosis.

Today, more surgeons believe that the opposite is true —that the more complete the *revascularization* (the more diseased arteries that are bypassed), the better the patient's chances are for complete and prolonged relief. Dr. Cooley says, "When multiple-bypass grafts are used, long-term results are improved, and re-operation for recurrent angina or heart failure or relief of symptoms is not often necessary." In fact, it is diffuse coronary artery disease that sometimes prevents the complete revascularization of blocked areas which is seen by Dr. Cooley as "the greatest risk factor."

However, most of the risks associated with bypass surgery are much lower than they used to be. For one thing, surgeons have become more experienced. They have acquired the skill needed to construct grafts to small, thin, delicate vessels and have learned more about how to keep patients stable during the operation. More is known about how to protect the heart during surgery and how to conserve the patient's blood during the operation, thus guarding against postoperative hemorrhaging.

The surgical techniques are remarkably similar in most hospitals and medical centers, but they differ considerably from methods used in the early days of bypass surgery. For instance, 92 percent of surgeons use *hypothermia* (a method of lowering body temperature by cooling the blood going from the heart-lung machine to the patient) and cold potassium *cardioplegia* (a solution that is injected into the aorta through a catheter which goes into the coronary arteries to preserve the store of energy in the myocardium during surgery) at 5 degrees centigrade to protect the heart during surgery. This permits the heart to remain in "cardiac arrest" (still) longer and more safely, thus allowing physicians the time to bypass small distal vessels if necessary, without risk of damage to the heart.

A report from the Montreal Heart Institute reveals that the mortality rate in older patients (aged sixty-five or older) dropped from 12 percent to 5 percent when the heart was protected by the use of cold cardioplegic solutions.

Careful monitoring after the operation has paralleled improved surgical techniques and has shortened the time a patient spends in the intensive-care unit. In 1980, nearly two-thirds of the patients in the Cleveland Clinic spent less than twenty-four hours in the intensive-care unit.

Because of improved blood-conservation methods, the

need for blood during surgery has decreased dramatically. In 1979, 58 percent of heart-bypass patients at the Cleveland Clinic received no blood during the operation. Dr. Floyd Loop says that as a result the incidence of hemorrhaging after surgery has been considerably reduced.

However, it is not only the immediate results of surgery that are important, but what happens five, ten, fifteen years later. There is concern about bypass grafts that do not remain open, and angina that returns and prompts the need for second or third operations. There has even been anxiety that the bypass operation itself may accelerate the process of atherosclerosis and hasten formation of new blockages. These developments have been called the "late results" of surgery.

Acceleration of Atherosclerosis

Early in the history of bypass surgery, a report in the *Journal of Thoracic Cardiovascular Surgery* suggested that the operation which was designed to open closed arteries actually helps to speed up the process of the disease. Since that time, there have been conflicting reports, not only about whether this is true, but also about how significant this progression is.

The theory is that bypass grafts may affect the native circulation—the natural flow of blood—by reducing it across the original coronary artery obstruction and by constricting the coronary artery.

A group at Johns Hopkins analyzed its own data and that of other institutions. It found that in 663 arteries that had been bypassed with grafts that were still open, there were 264 new blockages (40 percent). But in 727 arteries without grafts, there was only a new blockage rate of 6 percent. Because 85 percent of the new blockages of grafted arteries were near the graft, it was not considered likely that they represented the natural progression of the disease. It was suggested that they became blocked because of the surgery, not because of the normal course of atherosclerosis.

A study at the University of Alabama examined 121 patients' angiograms almost a year after surgery. New blockages and progression of pre-existing blockages were five times more frequent in grafted than in nongrafted arteries with similar initial disease. It did not matter if the bypass grafts were open or blocked—the new and progressive blockages occurred with similar frequency.

But the major randomized study done by the Veterans Administration did not find any "striking difference in the progression of the disease" between patients who received surgery and those who did not, when they were studied angiographically two years later. The report suggested that earlier studies may have yielded different results because those who participated in them were only patients who were having severe symptoms.

And a study at the Montreal Heart Institute, which examined patients angiographically one, three and six years after surgery, found little difference in the rate of progressive atherosclerosis between grafted and nongrafted arteries by the sixth year after the operation.

Nonetheless, Betty B., fifty-nine, who has had three operations for blocked arteries, is convinced that her problems have accelerated because she had surgery in the first place. Her first operation was in 1974, when she had a double bypass for blockages in her left anterior descending and right coronary arteries. "I went in because I was uncomfortable—not in extreme pain, but not able to be as active as I wanted," Betty says. "I guess I was naive, but no one ever told me that the operation wouldn't cure me. I thought I would go in, have this bypass and never have to worry again. And for two years, that seemed to be the case.

"Then I began getting these chest pains all over again. And this time they were worse than before. Another catheterization showed that there was more blockage in the right coronary artery. I think the doctor said it had increased from thirty-five percent to eighty-five percent. That's a lot in two years. Anyway, I had another operation. And again I was OK for a while. But the same thing happened. Pain. Shortness of breath. Worse than ever.

"I went back for another catheterization. The doctors all knew me by now. They called me by my first name. They said, 'Betty, what are you doing back here? You just can't stay away from us.'

"It turned out another blockage had increased. I don't even know which artery it was. I didn't care anymore. I just said, 'When can you operate?' "

Betty has the feeling that her disease was helped along by the first surgical procedure she had. She says if she knew then what she knows now, she would never have agreed to have it. Now she thinks she has no choice but will have to spend her life richocheting from one bypass operation to another.

Grafts That Do Not Remain Open

Patients suffering angina after bypass operations often do so because one or more of their grafts has not remained open (most grafts that will close do so within a few months after surgery). There is evidence that grafts to the left anterior descending artery remain patent (open) more frequently than do grafts to the circumflex or the right coronary arteries. And there are substantiated reports that grafts done with the internal mammary artery have a higher patency rate than grafts done with the saphenous leg vein.

Graft patency depends on many things:

· The year of the operation (those done in the early 1970s do not remain open as often or for as long as those done later);
· The rate of blood flow through the graft at the time of surgery;
· The diameter of the artery receiving the graft;
· The condition of the distal segment of the artery;
· Condition of the vein that is grafted (veins that have deteriorated before being grafted to the coronary artery and segments of the vein with pre-existing disease should not be used);
· The state of ventricular function (graft patency decreases in patients with poor ventricular function).

Dr. Favaloro says that rate of graft occlusion after the first year, in his experience, is about 1 to 2 percent annually.

The Cleveland Clinic reports that its vein-graft patency after twenty-two months is 84 percent, and of 609 patients with 891 grafts who were restudied four years after surgery, 82 percent of grafts were open. The patency rate is higher for internal mammary grafts—more than 95 percent.

A report from the Baylor College of Medicine on 250 patients followed for at least ten years showed that graft patency in 230, determined at a median follow-up of seven years, was 81.3 percent. Drs. Michael E. DeBakey and Gerald M. Lawrie say that "early concerns that saphenous vein grafts would often become obstructed ... have proved to be unfounded."

Dr. Loop says that he is using the internal mammary

artery more often even though it is more tedious to do. But there are advantages; namely, its increased patency.

Just as more complete revascularization of the heart seems to result in fewer deaths, it also contributes, say many physicians, to better patency rates.

Milwaukee's Dr. Dudley Johnson is perhaps the pioneer advocate for complete revascularization. He has done as many as eight bypasses on a patient. "When an operation has included many grafts," he says, "it is unlikely that all of them will close completely, and therefore the prognosis for the patient's longevity is improved."

Dr. Johnson has seen a steady increase in the average number of grafts required since he initiated the bypass operation in 1968. He evaluated 778 patients, who received 4 or more grafts, who had surgery between 1970 and 1975. Of this group, 598 patients received 4 grafts; 297 received 5; 65 received 6; 7 patients had 7 grafts; and 2 patients received 8. All major and secondary branches of the coronary system were used for bypass grafts. One to six years later, 49 of the patients had all bypasses open. And in no patient were all grafts closed. Dr. Johnson reports that no patient in the group needed a second operation.

The Texas Heart Institute in Houston also conducted a study from which it was concluded that a critical factor in the need for a second operation to relieve angina pain is the feasibility of complete revascularization the first time around.

Lesions that were considered not significant enough to bypass (50 to 70 percent blockages) turned out to be risk factors. Nine of ten unbypassed blockages progressed to significant occlusions within six months to four years after the initial operation. In five patients, this was the only reason for needing a second operation.

Dr. Floyd Loop of the Cleveland Clinic observes that

patients who require second operations for graft failure or progressive atherosclerosis seem to have a tendency toward premature coronary artery disease. For instance, at his clinic, the average age at the first operation was forty-nine, nearly ten years younger than the average patient who has bypass surgery. Fifty-one percent of these patients were operated on again solely for progressive disease in arteries that previously had not been grafted.

The surprising results of a study at the Medical College of Wisconsin, the Wood Veterans Administration Hospital and St. Luke's Hospital in Milwaukee reveal that the very risk factors that make one susceptible to atherosclerosis in the first place are often helpful in keeping grafts open. For instance, the study found a high correlation between graft patency soon after surgery and high diastolic blood pressure and higher cholesterol levels. Just as shocking was the finding that shorter, younger, lighter patients tended to have fewer grafts open than those who were heavier, stockier and older. Those with more disease before surgery also had more open grafts soon afterward. As if that were not enough, grafts in nonsmokers closed more frequently than they did in smokers.

The study's authors speculate that during the early postoperative stage, the blood flow in the heart may be more efficiently maintained at higher levels of blood pressure. And it may be that when arteries are obstructed, this induces the formation of collaterals (bypasses created by the body to compensate for the closed arteries) and thus increases potential blood flow beyond the obstruction. Since more cholesterol is associated with more disease, this may explain why higher cholesterol levels and graft patency seem related.

There was no explanation for the apparently higher incidence of new blockages in nonsmokers; and after the first year of follow-up, the relationship between high cholesterol and open grafts had vanished.

Despite grafts that close, an overwhelming number of patients who have bypass surgery experiences pain relief. What are the chances that it will continue?

The answer is difficult. There are two main reasons why angina pain returns: bypass grafts that have become closed; and the natural progression of atherosclerosis, which the surgery does not pretend to cure.

Most bypass grafts that will close do so in the first several months to a year following surgery. After that, the rate of closure is much lower. Reports claim figures from 3.5 to 13 percent a year.

However, the rate at which the disease progresses varies in each person. It may be that the bypass patient who stops smoking, cuts down on rich foods, engages in exercise and generally takes care of his/her body after surgery will experience slower progression (or even no progression) of the disease. On the other hand, persons who continue to gorge themselves on calorie-laden foods, fail to keep their blood pressure down and continue to smoke or work at high-pressure jobs may succumb faster. Or it may be that atherosclerosis, because it is genetically based, may march along on its own, regardless of any help it does or does not get from its victim.

A study by the Montreal Heart Institute and the University of Montreal concludes that "the effect of aortocoronary bypass graft surgery is transient in a high proportion of patients and that deterioration of results is related to late graft modifications and progression of atherosclerosis, particularly in ungrafted coronary arteries."

Another study by the same institute, released in January 1981, made intriguing revelations. Of 224 patients studied over a five-year period, 129 had complete or partial relief of angina. In 97 patients, the improvement was retained for up to five years, but in 32 patients the initial improvement deteriorated after the first year.

What made the difference between the two groups? Smoking, age, sex, severity of angina before surgery, the number of arteries involved and even the critical ejection fraction did *not* seem to have a bearing. However, there were characteristics that were significantly different in those who sustained pain relief and those who did not. Those whose pain returned had had abnormalities on their resting electrocardiograms before surgery, had elevated cholesterol and triglyceride levels before surgery and had failed to receive complete revascularizations, meaning that they were left with blockages that had not been bypassed. When all factors were present, the frequency of improvement loss was 42.9 percent.

When some patients were given angiograms after surgery, it was found that among those who had recurrent angina, grafts had either closed or the disease had progressed.

Dr. Lucien Campeau and Dr. Martial G. Bourassa and their associates who reported the study conclude that, "Bypass surgery is currently considered a palliative therapy. It appears that recurrence of angina after the operation is related to the development or progression of obstructive disease in the grafts and in the coronary arteries, most likely caused by atherosclerosis. Thus, it seems reasonable to assume that risk factors known to promote atherosclerosis are also probably involved."

In that case, will patients improve if they have second operations?

The rate of success in terms of relief of pain is usually considerably less after the second operation than after the first, concludes Dr. Donald C. Wukasch and his colleagues at the Texas Heart Institute. Ninety percent of people had relief of pain after the first operation, but only 63 percent improved after the second. Re-operating was not helpful for treatment of cardiac failure; even if patients were relieved of angina, they remained incapacitated because of congestive heart failure.

However, a report from the Cleveland Clinic indicates that 89 percent of patients are alive five years after the second operation. While second operations are technically more difficult to do, the mortality rate and risk of heart attack is no greater than it is for the first surgery. But in the group of patients studied by Dr. Wukasch and his associates, there was a greater risk of hemorrhage, and more blood transfusions were required.

In summary, patients undergoing heart-bypass surgery today can expect successful results because of new advances in surgery. There is still some risk, but Dr. Loop says it is lower than it would be for a patient who has atherosclerosis and is undergoing a gall bladder operation.

The most significant risk factors are probably the state of the left ventricle, the extent of the disease and the age of the patient. But a five-year study of 1,718 patients from the Medical College of Wisconsin is also worth looking at. It cites cholesterol level as an important risk factor in determining survival from bypass surgery after five years.

The findings show that survival was significantly lower for patients who:

- Had many arteries blocked (twice the mortality of patients with less blockages);
- Were older than fifty;
- Had seriously impaired left ventricular function (three times the five-year mortality rate of other surgical patients);
- Had left ventricular end-diastolic pressure (see Chapter 3) greater than 18;

· Had a cholesterol level of 350 or more;
· Had had more than one heart attack prior to operation.

Patients with history of stroke had a five-year survival rate of only 32.4 percent, and patients with systolic blood pressure greater than 150 had poorer survival rates than those with readings below 150. However, there was no significant association between survival rate and triglyceride level, diastolic blood pressure, height, weight, incidence of diabetes or smoking.

The researchers were able to predict the probability of surviving five years after surgery. For instance, they cite the case of a fifty-five-year-old man with severely impaired left ventricular function, a poor left ventricular end-diastolic pressure (see Chapter 3), a moderate degree of arterial blockage and a cholesterol level of 265. This man would have an 80 percent chance of surviving five years after surgery. But a similar man, with all of his arteries almost totally blocked, would have only a 63 percent chance of surviving five years after surgery.

The authors of this study, headed by Dr. Raymond G. Hoffmann, observe that the information they have amassed should "facilitate patient education about the expected results of surgery, and thus the decision for or against surgery will be made by a better-informed patient."

The "better-informed" patient is often more puzzled than the less-informed one. He or she knows that the skill of the surgeon is critical and that the hospital or medical center where the operation is performed can make a difference in life or death. It is this patient who is often experiencing mixed emotions: Shall I travel a long distance to be operated on by a "superstar"? Or should I stay closer to home where I can be near my family and friends? Do most medical centers have competent cardiac surgeons? Shall I depend on my cardiologist's recommendations?

The choice is not easy. The country has hundreds of competent cardiac surgeons experienced in bypass surgery. In 1979, the mean case load was 137 bypass operations per surgeon, and only 46 surgeons (in a survey conducted by Dr. Donald W. Miller, Jr., and associates) did fewer than 25 that year. Less than 25 percent of the operations was done in university or federal hospitals; the majority was performed in private hospitals or medical centers by surgical specialists.

Anyone considering bypass surgery should not hesitate to ask the surgeon he is thinking of using tough, direct questions, as suggested by Wisconsin's Dr. Johnson:

- How many bypass operations have you done last year?
- What is your mortality rate?
- How many of your patients had other heart problems that needed attention in addition to bypass?
- How many of your patients had a poor heart muscle (which makes surgery more complicated)?
- How many of your patients suffered a heart attack during the operation? How many suffered a stroke?
- What kind of grafts do you use—leg vein or mammary artery?
- How many of your grafts stay open?
- What is *my* risk, based on what you know about my history and my coronary anatomy?

And it is important to remember that the surgical mortality cited by any medical center or any doctor must be considered in relationship to the seriousness of the heart cases included in those statistics. For instance, some hospitals and some surgeons will perform surgery only on patients with normal or slightly abnormal left ventricles. Others will not handle patients with widespread disease.

Their mortality statistics may look better than those from centers which do operations on more seriously ill persons.

A report called "Optimal Resources for Cardiac Surgery" which appeared in *Circulation* magazine concludes that the following are necessary to ensure the best possible surgical results:

· A well-staffed operating room;
· Intensive-care units with advanced technical equipment and skilled nurses on duty twenty-four hours a day;
· A work load per doctor that permits him or her to operate on large numbers of patients, but which does not prevent him or her from developing his or her clinical skills and engaging in research;
· Skilled nursing staff;
· Qualified anesthesiology staff;
· Complete diagnostic facilities, including a catheterization laboratory, blood bank and pulmonary function unit.

The report, prepared by the Inter-Society Commission for Heart Disease Resources, emphasizes that the smallest number of operations that would qualify an institution to do bypass surgery would be four to six such operations a week. There should be at least two, preferably three, qualified cardiac surgeons, two senior surgical residents and a minimum of four junior residents in the hospital.

The final decision must be made by the patient. Leonard Tose, owner of the Philadelphia Eagles football team, chose to fly to Texas and have his surgery (heart-valve replacement) done by Dr. Denton Cooley. Others will rely on their cardiologists, in whom they have trust and faith, to make suitable recommendations. Still others will ask friends and relatives who have had the operation how they felt about their surgeons.

"In the end, after all the questions and all the recommendations, it turns out to be a 'gut decision,' " says Shelly T., a forty-eight-year-old woman who underwent the operation four years ago. "I saw three different surgeons and finally chose the one with whom I felt comfortable. I knew he had an excellent reputation, and I talked with people whose operations he had done. But what impressed me most was his manner. He treated me like a person. He answered my questions patiently, and he made me feel comfortable. I had faith in him. I trusted that he would make me well."

He did. Shelly has had no trouble since her operation in June 1977.

6 CAN ANGINA BE TREATED WITHOUT SURGERY?

When Michael Z., a forty-four-year-old California businessman, had his first experience with angina, it was December 1965, before the bypass operation was in common use. Michael remembers that he was stunned by a feeling of pressure in his chest as he was paneling the recreation room of his new redwood and glass home in Beverly Hills.

But the pain he felt was brief, and when he rested for a few minutes, it vanished as mysteriously as it had come. Michael forgot about it until several days later, when he experienced it again. This time it happened while he was playing tennis.

Michael couldn't understand it. He had always been in good health, had never been in a hospital; in fact, Michael couldn't remember the last time he had seen a doctor. It had been at least seven or eight years.

He made an appointment with his wife's physician, an internist, who gave him a complete physical examination; asked him dozens of questions; sent him for a chest X ray, electrocardiogram, blood tests and a urinalysis.

Michael's family history of heart disease was negative, except for an uncle who had had a heart attack three years earlier and had recovered. But Michael's physical examination gave the doctor cause for concern. His blood pres-

sure was 180/104, an elevation of both the systolic and
diastolic pressures. His cholesterol level was 310, above
normal. His triglyceride level was a whopping 450. And
Michael was about twenty pounds overweight.

From their conversation, the doctor was able to tell that
Michael was a hard-driving, impatient, ambitious person,
who became easily agitated and frustrated.

Michael and his doctor had a long talk that day. The
doctor told him that the pains he was experiencing
sounded like classic angina, but that there was medication
he thought would help. He told Michael that he had a
number of other problems that could be ominous, and
that it would be crucial for Michael to alter his life-style
enough so that they could be modified.

Most important, he told Michael that the success of the
treatment prescribed would depend largely on Michael's
willingness to comply with it. The physician was concerned that Michael would not be sufficiently motivated
to adhere to the treatment program.

His program, a medical approach to angina, included:

- Lowering Michael's blood pressure. He prescribed
  medication, a diuretic at first, that he hoped would
  bring results. He also told Michael to eat a banana or
  orange each day to replenish the potassium that would
  be depleted from his body as a result of taking the
  diuretic. Michael was to return in a week to have his
  pressure checked again.
- Placing Michael on a diet that would lower his weight,
  his cholesterol and triglyceride levels. Michael was
  told to cut down on fats, limit his consumption of red
  meat to twice a week, cut down on fresh fruit (because
  of the tendency of fresh fruit to raise triglyceride levels) and reduce his intake of foods containing sugar
  and salt.

- Prescribing nitroglycerin, which has been the traditional method of treating angina for the last century and is still used today, often with excellent results. Nitroglycerin works by decreasing the work of the heart and improving ventricular function. It permits the heart to work under less resistance, and it dilates the coronary arteries. Michael was told to place the nitroglycerin (which comes in a tiny white tablet) under his tongue and let it dissolve whenever he felt chest pain. He was also advised to take nitroglycerin prophylactically; if he knew, for instance, that playing tennis was likely to bring on pain, he should take the nitroglycerin before he started a game. A small dose was prescribed initially. Michael was told that the drug would probably not have significant side effects, that it is not habit forming and that its potency does not decrease with continued use. Side effects, if they appeared, could be headache or a burning sensation of the tongue.
- Encouraging Michael to learn how to relax and reduce his anxiety level. Among the doctor's suggestions were frequent brief vacations, medication, working shorter hours and learning how to delegate responsibility.

Michael admits that at first he didn't take his doctor's warnings seriously. After all, he felt well except for the occasional angina, and even that wasn't incapacitating, just a nuisance. But within three or four months, the angina pain worsened. His nitroglycerin had to be increased. And then Michael's best friend, a man he had known for fifteen years—a man who, like Michael, had never been ill—died suddenly from cardiac causes.

"That sobered me," says Michael. "From that point on, I was scared, and I got serious about losing the weight and

taking the blood-pressure medicine and not driving myself so hard."

Today, Michael is sixty. He still has angina but says it is
less severe now. When he does get the pain, he takes his
nitroglycerin. He has never needed other medication. His
blood pressure is down to 140/82, and he has shed 21
pounds since 1964. His cholesterol level varies, but he
generally maintains it at about 225. He no longer eats
desserts, and his triglyceride level is 175, a big drop.

Michael's physician considers his angina stable. His
electrocardiograms continue to be normal. Unless there is
a change in Michael's condition, the physician does not
expect him to be a candidate for coronary artery surgery.

If Michael had experienced angina for the first time in
1978 instead of 1964, the approach to his condition may
have been different, depending on the physician he consulted. Since many doctors consider any new angina to be
"unstable" angina, it is likely that Michael may have been
whisked to the catheterization laboratory. If his blockages
were significant enough, surgery may have been recommended. There would have been no opportunity to learn
whether Michael's "unstable" angina, if treated medically, would have become "stable."

"The trouble is that for some patients medical treatment is more difficult than surgery," says Duke University's Dr. Robert Rosati. "It is easier for patients to say, 'Fix
me up so I don't have to take that medicine.' But we have
the responsibility to encourage people to take better care
of themselves."

Today, medical management of angina is practiced
mainly when:

· Coronary artery disease is not advanced or disabling
  enough to warrant surgery;
· Atherosclerosis is too severe (there is too much disease

in distal vessels, perhaps accompanied by poor ventricular function) to permit surgery;
· The patient has other risk factors that would make surgery unwise, conditions such as severe kidney disease, vascular disease in the brain or extremities, or advanced cancer;
· The patient refuses to have surgery, although he or she is considered a candidate and the physician has indeed recommended it.

As in Michael's case, medical care involves attention to conditions that influence atherosclerosis and may need correction. These include hypertension, diabetes, high levels of cholesterol and triglycerides, introduction of appropriate exercise, reduction of stress and cessation of smoking. But unlike Michael, many patients are haphazard about their adherence to all or parts of their treatment program.

"What we are concerned about is whether the patient will adhere to the treatment we have prescribed, and this is a tremendous responsibility," says Philadelphia cardiologist, Dr. Robert Katz. "Any medical regimen is only as good as the compliance of the patient in following it. Especially if the medical regimen is a rigid one, there is a tendency for patients not to adhere."

Especially for men and women who are not in a lot of discomfort, there is a tendency to become lax about such aspects of their treatment as regular exercise and reducing stress. They skip their high-blood-pressure medication, continue to smoke and gorge themselves on forbidden foods.

Dr. Katz agrees that it is easier to send someone to surgery. "That way you can feel as though you are really doing something—you are sending the patient to get his disease cut out. But in this kind of disease, which is progressive, you can't ever really do that. Still, recommending surgery is doing something concrete.

"When you don't send a patient to surgery, you are always a little uneasy that something might happen. And the medical treatment becomes a shared responsibility between the physician and the patient. The patient and the doctor must understand each other, and medication and other treatment must be tailored to the patient's lifestyle."

Most cardiologists agree that patient adherence varies; that physicians cannot assume that patients are following the prescribed medical regimen, even if they say they are. "Patients want to please their doctors, so sometimes they lie," Dr. Katz says. "Doctors must take this into account."

While many patients are remiss about taking medicine for high blood pressure (because the condition causes them no discomfort), will not give up smoking, are unable or unwilling to alter their life-styles, a majority *will* take medication when needed to relieve the pain of angina. There are a number of medications that help.

Nitroglycerin: Most angina patients will begin with nitroglycerin, especially if the angina is mild. This is the tablet that Michael, the first patient described, places under his tongue when he gets chest pain or is about to engage in an activity that may precipitate his angina. Michael uses the tablet before tennis, sex and conferences with his employer.

Dr. Willis Hurst of Emory University says it is crucial to instruct a patient in the use of nitroglycerin. It should be taken, he says, whenever the patient feels chest distress. The distress does not have to be pain but may be pressure, tightness, burning, shortness of breath or whatever it is that brings on discomfort. If nitroglycerin is not effective, it is usually because the discomfort is not associated with the heart. However, it may indicate that the distress is

more than angina, that it represents more serious ischemia (oxygen deficiency, usually caused by a blocked
blood vessel) or that it may be associated with a condition
that is made worse by nitroglycerin (an example is *hypertrophic cardiomyopathy*, a condition in which blood flow
from the left ventricle is obstructed). Sometimes the medication does not bring relief because it has lost its potency.
The patient can usually tell because the tablet will not
burn under the tongue.

In addition to headache, which a few patients experience, occasionally a person may develop a syndrome characterized by coldness, clamminess and profuse sweating.
Sometimes an individual with these symptoms is thought
to be suffering from a heart attack; but when this diagnosis
cannot be confirmed, a sensitivity to nitroglycerin may be
isolated as the cause.

Long-Acting Nitrates: Long-acting nitrates, which
can be administered in the form of ointment to the skin
or orally, can improve the functioning of the heart, reduce the oxygen the heart requires and help coronary
circulation. These nitrates are used in anticipation of the
occurrence of angina. Nitroglycerin ointment, for instance, may be applied to the skin, on any part of the
body, at night to prevent nocturnal angina or during the
day before a game of golf or handball. A commonly used
long-acting nitrate (which can be swallowed or chewed)
is isosorbide.

It is important that long-acting nitrates be administered
in the appropriate dosage to be effective. For example,
Dr. Katz says that 10 mg. of isosorbide four times a day
may be worthless; but 40 mg. every four hours with two
inches of paste (nitroglycerin ointment) applied to the
skin could be extremely effective.

Beta-Blockers: Emory's Dr. Hurst believes that beta-
blocking agents "are the greatest advance in the treat-

ment of angina pectoris since nitrates were introduced one hundred years ago." In this country, beta-blockers began to come into general usage in the late 1960s, but it was not until the early 1970s that they were distributed to patients on a widespread basis. Dr. Hurst believes that new calcium antagonists (described later in this chapter) offer much promise also.

Beta-blockers work by decreasing the heart rate and reducing the amount of oxygen the heart muscle needs. Sometimes they raise left ventricular end-diastolic pressure (see Chapter 3) and have an antiarrhythmic effect on the heart. Often they are used in conjunction with nitrates in doses (from 10 mg. to 1 gram) that will help prevent angina, and they are usually introduced along with nitroglycerin. Most physicians will not wait until nitrates have been tried first before prescribing a beta-blocker. The most commonly used beta-blocker in this country is propranolol (also known as Inderal), and most people require doses of 80 to 320 mg. a day to obtain comfort. It may take up to a week before improvement in angina is noticed. Patients must be warned by their physicians not to suddenly discontinue the use of propranolol, since it can cause an increase in angina symptoms or may even precipitate a heart attack.

Side effects occur more often with beta-blockers than they do with nitrates and may include fatigue, depression, weakness, diarrhea, amnesia, hallucinations, heart failure, decreased sexual performance and precipitation of asthma in susceptible persons. Often, however, these symptoms will lessen as the patient becomes accustomed to the drug. Some studies have shown that 85 percent of patients have at least a 50 percent reduction of angina if they are given adequate dosages of propranolol.

Dr. Harold L. Rutenberg, clinical associate professor of medicine and former chairman of the department of cardiology at Pennsylvania Hospital, feels strongly that the side effects of beta-blockers have been seriously overemphasized. "In my personal experience, they are among the safest medications that I have ever prescribed," he says.

Other beta-blockers include practolol, tolamolol, oxprenolol and alprenolol, and for those whose symptoms are not relieved with propranolol, one of the others is often effective.

Not only are beta-blockers successful in relieving angina, many studies indicate that they have a positive effect on the incidence of heart attack. In fact, in October, 1981, the National Heart, Lung, and Blood Institutes of the National Institutes of Health halted a nationwide project to test the effectiveness of propranolol (Inderal) in reducing mortality after heart attack. The testing was stopped because it became clear, nine months before the study was to have been completed, that the drug was indeed effective.

The study was a large one, including 3,837 men and women between thirty and sixty who had had a heart attack. Those enrolled were assigned at random to two groups—one receiving propranolol and the other receiving a placebo. The drug was started, beginning five to twenty-one days after the heart attack and was given, in substantial doses, for periods up to thirty months.

Results showed that the patients who received propranolol had a 26 percent lower mortality than the group that did not, the greatest difference coming in the first year after the heart attack. It is not known whether the drug would be effective if it were begun months or years after a person has had a heart attack.

And in November, 1981, the Food and Drug Administration approved the drug timolol, another beta-blocker, which it says can reduce by one third the chances of a second heart attack. The FDA's approval came shortly after the results of a large-scale study done in Norway were reported in the New England Journal of Medicine. The study suggested that patients who have had heart attacks are at a 40 percent lower risk of having another one if treated with timolol. The death rate of heart-attack patients considered to be at high risk (see Chapter 4) was slashed almost in half when the drug was used.

The study included 1,884 patients from twenty Norwegian hospitals and was conducted over three years. The drug was given in the form of a tablet to some patients one to four weeks after the heart attack. Other patients received a placebo. In the three-year follow-up period, there were 152 deaths among those who took the placebo, but only 98 among those who received timolol. Risk factors of the patients, such as age, sex, smoking habits, high blood pressure or location or extent of the previous heart attack, did not affect the outcome. Of fifteen other studies with four beta-blockers (propranolol, practolol, alprenolol and oxprenolol), four demonstrated a reduction in mortality from heart attack. The studies were all performed on persons who had had a previous myocardial infarction. In eleven of the studies, the beta-blocking drugs were begun within the first two days after the heart attack; only one study showed a reduction in mortality. The drug used was propranolol.

In the other four studies, beta-blockers were not started until two or more weeks after the initial heart attack and were continued for up to thirty-six months. Three of these studies demonstrated significant reductions in mortality; the drugs used were practolol and alprenolol.

There are two other important studies which tested the reactions of patients who had suffered heart attacks and were subsequently treated with beta-blockers. A multi-center study conducted in forty-nine hospitals in the

United Kingdom, Italy and Yugoslavia did not find any significant difference in the rate of heart attack between a control group of patients receiving a placebo and a group receiving 40 mg. of propranolol three times a day. All persons participating in the study had had a previous heart attack involving the anterior wall of the heart.

The study worked this way. There were 720 patients, aged seventy or less, who entered the study from two to fourteen days after they had suffered a heart attack. They were given either propranolol or a placebo three times a day. Follow-ups were done at one, three, six and nine months. However, persons who developed angina following the heart attack had to be eliminated from the study, since they required beta-blockers and could not be randomized into groupings that might prevent them from receiving them.

The two groups—the one receiving a placebo and the one receiving propranolol—were similar in characteristics. For instance, the mean age of the patients on placebo was 54.8, and of the patients on propranolol it was 55. The mean weight and height were similar, and the number of smokers was the same. Fifteen of those receiving placebos had hypertension, as did thirteen of those receiving the beta-blocker. Forty percent of those in the placebo group had angina, compared with 35 percent of the group receiving propranolol.

It was hoped that the results might show a 50 percent reduction in mortality in the group receiving propranolol, but this result was not demonstrated. In fact, the difference in mortality rates between the two groups was not statistically significant. And the rate of nonfatal subsequent heart attack was also similar in both groups.

In this study, there were several factors that seemed to bear on whether the patient would have a second heart attack, but the method of treatment was not one of them.

The characteristics that made a definite difference were age (older persons being at higher risk), heart rate and arrhythmias of the heart at the time of entrance into the study. Characteristics which may have had an influence were sex (females doing more poorly than males), history of smoking and history of heart attack.

However, the investigators admit that their sample was small, and it is possible that the use of propranolol may produce a reduction in mortality that is less than 50 percent, the hypothesis upon which this trial was based.

Another multicenter international study, begun in 1972, did show the effectiveness of the beta-blocker practolol in improving the prognosis of myocardial infarction.

Here, 3,038 patients from sixty-seven hospitals and medical centers recovering from acute heart attacks were entered into a study that began one to four weeks after the attack. Follow-up took place at one, six and twelve months. The theory was that the use of beta-blocking agents, in appropriate dosages, administered to patients who survived heart attacks might reduce mortality by reducing the incidence of arrhythmias. It is known that sudden death after heart attack is caused mainly by arrhythmias.

The patients were randomized into two groups: one which received a 100 mg. tablet of practolol; and the other which received a similar-looking tablet that was a placebo. The test was double-blind, which meant that no one (not even doctors or nurses) knew who was receiving which tablet. A sealed copy of the identity of the tablet was sent to each hospital pharmacist and physician in the event of an emergency which required knowing which tablet a particular patient was taking.

Both groups were similar in characteristics. The mean age was fifty-five, 36 percent of each group had had previous angina, there was a similar number of smokers in each group and the mean systolic and diastolic blood pressure was the same.

There was a significant difference in the numbers of cardiac deaths between the two groups—forty-seven with patients on practolol and seventy-three with patients receiving a placebo. Of those receiving the beta-blocker, sixty-nine suffered nonfatal heart attack within the year, while eighty-nine of those receiving placebos had infarctions within twelve months.

As in the study with propranolol, the characteristics of each patient when he or she entered the study were important. The three factors that seemed to influence what happened to patients in relation to their treatment were their body size, the site of the original heart attack (which part of the heart was affected) and the level of diastolic blood pressure.

For instance, in patients whose heart attack had been in the anterior (front) part of the heart, the number of deaths among patients taking practolol was less than half that of the group taking the placebo. However, when patients had their heart attacks in the inferior (lower) part of the heart, there was no reduction in mortality among those taking practolol. The number of sudden deaths was, however, reduced.

When diastolic blood pressure was 78 or below, patients taking practolol had better survival rates. There were fifteen deaths among those on the beta-blocker, and thirty-six among those on the placebo. It was interesting that the greatest difference in mortality was shown between the group of patients with an anterior heart attack and blood pressure below 78. Among these persons, there were only five deaths in the beta-blocker group and twenty-six in the placebo group. However, those who had had heart attacks of the inferior part of the heart showed no decrease in death, no matter the level of diastolic pressure when they entered the study. Lightweight persons also did better than heavier persons, perhaps because of the relationship between body weight and the blood level of the beta-blocker.

The conclusions of the trial, published in the *British Medical Journal* in 1975, were that "patients should receive long-term beta-adrenoreceptor blocking treatment after anterior myocardial infarction unless specific contraindications exist. Treatment should probably be initiated as soon as the doctor is satisfied that there is no serious impairment of conduction and no immediate prospect of congestive heart failure." Pennsylvania Hospital's Dr. Harold Rutenberg cautions that "comparisons between groups studied are only valid when patients are matched for myocardial function [ejection fraction, history of heart failure, heart size, etc.] since this is the most important prognostic indicator in coronary heart disease."

Digitalis: The efficacy of using digitalis in treating coronary heart disease is far from settled. Some physicians think it can aggravate angina because it increases the force of heart contractions and elevates the level of oxygen needed by the heart. And there is no question that certain doses of digitalis can produce heart arrhythmias and, in some patients, can cause premature ventricular beats. However, under certain conditions it may relieve arrhythmias, which may be present in some people who also have angina. But there is no evidence that the use of digitalis benefits people who have angina. Emory's Dr. Willis Hurst believes that digitalis can be tried to manage angina with special subsets of patients, including those who have angina at night, those who have progressive angina, those with enlarged hearts or pulmonary congestion. He does not advise digitalis routinely for patients who have had an acute heart attack because it could aggravate the condition, but he may use it in specific patients with certain characteristics, particularly where heart failure may be involved.

Because there is increasing data that correlates the level of lipids (fats) in the blood to coronary artery disease, some physicians will prescribe "lipid-lowering" drugs to patients whose blood tests show that they are high in cholesterol and/or triglycerides. However, other physicians prefer to treat this condition nutritionally by lowering the amount of fats consumed.

A study by Drs. David T. Nash, clinical professor of medicine, Goeffredo Gensini and Paulo Esente of the Upstate Medical Center and the St. Joseph's Hospital and Health Center in Syracuse, New York, looked at the effects of lowering blood lipid levels in the *progression* and *regression* of coronary artery disease.

Their research involved twenty-five patients, all of whom had had angiograms showing coronary artery disease. All of the patients had more than a 50 percent blockage of a major coronary artery, and all had a cholesterol level of 250 or more. Every patient received colestipol, a lipid-lowering drug, twice a day. After a month, those whose cholesterol had dropped at least 15 percent were placed in a treatment group that was to continue with the drug for two years. Those patients who had less than a 15 percent cholesterol reduction were separated into another group and given a placebo.

After two months, the patients taking colestipol whose level of triglycerides was below 200 or who had shown an additional 5 percent drop in cholesterol had their dose of the medication increased. After three months, these patients were given another lipid-lowering drug—clofibrate. The patients who exhibited an additional 5 percent drop in cholesterol or a 15 percent or more drop in triglycerides continued to receive both drugs—colestipol and clofibrate. But if there was no additional reduction in blood lipids, clofibrate was stopped and only colestipol was given.

The patients who, after one month on colestipol, had a triglyceride level of more than 200 had 1.0 gram of clofibrate twice a day added to their regimen. A month later, the colestipol dosage was increased.

Of the original patients studied, thirteen received lipid-lowering drugs (thirteen took colestipol and clofibrate, and one took only colestipol), and twelve were maintained on a placebo after having taken colestipol for one month.

Patients in both groups were placed on a low cholesterol diet. Every month for the first six months, and every two months thereafter, the patients were re-examined and blood lipid levels were taken. At the end of two years, all patients received angiograms again.

The physicians who interpreted the angiograms did not know which therapy the patient had received, nor did they have any information about the patient's blood lipid level.

When the angiograms taken before and after medical treatment were compared, this is what they showed:

·   Two of the thirteen patients treated on lipid-lowering agents showed *regression* of their blockages, and the other eleven remained *stable.*
·   Of the twelve patients treated with placebos, seven showed *progression,* four remained *stable* and one showed *regression.*

The doctors point out that both groups—those receiving the lipid-lowering drugs and those receiving placebos—were similar in a variety of risk factors, which included sex, age, smoking history, family history, hypertension, obesity, diabetes, Type A personality and previous history of open-heart surgery. There was an equal number of patients with multiple-vessel disease in each group.

The patients who showed *regression* of their blockages had fewer risks, but the number of risks did not seem to account for whether patients remained stable or progressed in the severity of their clogged arteries.

And patients who experienced reduction in blockages were those whose blood lipids were more dramatically reduced.

Studies such as this one are not easy to duplicate because they involve subjecting patients to invasive procedures (angiograms) which carry risk although minimal. Many patients are unwilling to take part in such research. Nonetheless, the authors of this study believe the results should encourage other investigators to verify or refute the significant findings.

Calcium Antagonists: A group of drugs known as calcium antagonists has been shown to eliminate or substantially reduce pain in patients suffering from chronic stable angina. The drugs have been marketed for several years in other countries, such as Italy, England and Germany, as an effective treatment for angina, and by the time this book is printed, they will probably be on the market in the United States. Verapamil, administered intravenously, has already been approved to treat arrhythmias. Calcium antagonists include perhexiline, diltiazem, verapamil, nifedipine and lidoflazine.

They work by blocking the uptake of calcium by the myocardial cells, by dilating coronary arteries and by dilating peripheral arteries. This lowers blood pressure and reduces a phenomenon that physicians refer to as *afterload.* Afterload is the pressure against which the heart has to pump when it first starts to contract.

While this class of drugs has been amazingly helpful to patients who suffer from Prinzmetal's or *variant angina* (angina caused by spasm), there has been less evidence that it is as useful for men and women who have atherosclerosis.

However, new, albeit limited, research is suggesting that coronary artery disease, too, may be responsive to calcium antagonists.

A study conducted on fifteen patients with typical angina, verified by a positive stress test, showed a 15 to 25 percent improvement in exercise tolerance after the patients had been treated with diltiazem. Other studies, published in this country and in Europe, which compared patients on verapamil and nifedipine with those on a placebo showed an even greater improvement in exercise tolerance—20 to 25 percent.

Research by Evelund and Oro compared the effect of beta-blockers (such as propranolol) with calcium antagonists. In this study, patients initially took a beta-blocker for three weeks. During the next three weeks, they were randomly given either a placebo or nifedipine. For the next week, they were switched to the other medication. During the final three weeks, everyone took both medications.

Results showed a 17 percent improvement in exercise tolerance with patients who were on beta-blockers, a 21 percent improvement on nifedipine and a 42 percent improvement during the last three weeks of the trial, where a combination of nifedipine and beta-blocker was used.

The National Heart, Lung, and Blood Institute also conducted a study with verapamil on eleven male patients with coronary artery disease (documented by angiograms) and angina experienced on exertion, who were followed at or referred to the Institute's cardiology branch. Patients selected to participate were those who continued to have angina, despite having taken doses of propranolol designed to relieve their chest pain (doses ranging from 160 mg. to 320 mg. a day). Seven of the eleven men were in Functional Class III, and four were in Functional Class IV, as established by the New York Heart Association (see Chapter 1). Five had had prior heart attacks, one had congestive heart failure and five had already had bypass surgery.

Some patients were treated for a period of forty-eight hours with verapamil, others with propranolol and the others with a placebo. After each drug, there was a twenty-four-hour rest period during which no medication was administered. Then each patient was switched to a different drug.

When this part of the study was completed, patients were treated with a combination of propranolol and increasing doses of verapamil.

All patients were stress-tested after each medication or combination of medications was stopped. Results showed that ten of the eleven men were able to pedal at least one minute longer on the bicycle after they had taken verapamil (480 mg. per day), and seven were able to increase their exercise performance. The "best dose" of propranolol (the dose that seemed to work best for the patient) improved the duration of exercise by at least one minute in five men, and two of those were able to increase their exercise tolerance.

But it was the combination of verapamil with the best dose of propranolol that brought the most gratifying results. Here, ten of the eleven patients demonstrated exercise improvement, and exercise duration was increased in eight patients. In nine of the eleven patients, angina did not occur at all during the exercise.

Not only do calcium antagonists work as well or better

than beta-blockers for many people, they seem to have fewer side effects.

Additional advantages are that:

· They increase coronary blood flow, while beta-blockers may decrease it.
· They may prevent spasm of the arteries.
· They can be used in patients who have chronic obstructive pulmonary disease.
· Based on animal research, they may reduce the size of a heart attack and may prevent ventricular fibrillation (arrhythmias) induced by ischemic heart disease. (Propranolol, too, may reduce size of heart attack)

In 1973, a study was initiated at Stanford University Medical Center to determine the effect of calcium antagonists on patients with unstable angina caused by coronary artery disease.

Results of the study indicated that spasms of the coronary artery superimposed on severe coronary disease occurred frequently in patients with unstable angina. Therefore, a calcium antagonist might be ideally suited for therapy for this kind of patient. Dr. John Speer Schroeder, associate professor of clinical medicine and cardiology at Stanford University Medical Center, points out that because the course of unstable angina is so unpredictable, it is difficult to conduct clinical trials to test the effectiveness of a specific drug. "However, non-controlled studies [studies where there is not a control group of patients receiving a placebo while another group is receiving the test drug, but where all patients are receiving the test drug] show that diltiazem, nifedipine and verapamil are highly effective for unstable angina pectoris and will become the therapy of choice," he says.

Dr. Attilio Maseri, a professor at the University of Lon-

don's Royal Postgraduate Medical School, has been studying calcium antagonists for a long time. During a 1980
visit to the United States, Dr. Maseri suggested that many
of the coronary bypass operations performed in America
could be avoided if patients were treated with calcium
antagonists (sometimes called slow calcium channel
blockers). Dr. Maseri says that while narrowed arteries
that eventually block blood flow to the heart are responsible for some heart attacks, another "major culprit in ini-
tiating the chain of events leading to heart attack is
spasms that constrict vessels that are clogged, as well as
those that are not."

However, many physicians argue that, based on angiographic studies, patients who receive surgery are those
who have clogged vessels, not coronary artery spasm.
Some of them may have spasm superimposed on the artery blockages, but the obstructions are present and often
require bypass surgery to reroute blood flow to the heart.

"I believe that spasm plays a role in the genesis of
angina pectoris," says Dr. Isadore Rosenfeld, clinical professor of medicine at the New York Hospital–Cornell
Medical Center, and the author of Second Opinion. "The
extent of the phenomenon has not yet been documented,
but it exists. Spasm, when it occurs, is almost always
superimposed on underlying obstructive disease," Dr.
Rosenfeld says. "When one operates on these people—
even after relieving the obstruction—they may still have
angina, by virtue of the pre-existing spasm. Indeed, such
coronary artery spasm may produce symptoms, on occa-
sion, in individuals with completely 'clean' coronary arteries. If such patients are tried on the calcium blockers,
this may reduce the need for bypass, at least temporarily,
in a certain number."

Dr. Schroeder suggests that beta-blockers may be on
the way out for use in treating patients with stable angina

if calcium antagonists prove to be as effective and as free of significant side effects as is so far indicated.

There have been reports on other drugs that seem to be helpful in preventing heart attack, but they are not yet routinely used, even for patients who have experienced a previous heart attack. And there is no evidence yet that they can relieve pain in patients suffering from angina caused by atherosclerosis. However, since the clinical course of coronary artery disease includes heart attack, a patient's prognosis is likely to improve if he or she can avoid having one.

Streptokinase: This therapy is not being used to treat angina, but it has been used to stop a heart attack if the patient can reach the hospital quickly. When a blood clot forms in a clogged artery and blocks the flow of blood to the heart, the portions of the heart muscle that are denied oxygen die. But if the clot can be broken up within six hours after chest pain begins, it can stop the attack and preserve the heart muscle. Streptokinase is injected into the coronary artery through a tube inserted in the groin, which snakes its way up into the artery and dissolves the clot. The procedure only takes two or three hours; but since the episode is a warning that there is blockage in the coronary arteries, a coronary angiogram and possible surgery are often necessary.

Anturane: This is a drug which has been licensed by the Food and Drug Administration for almost a quarter of a century as a remedy against gout. But although a major study several years ago showed Anturane to be effective in preventing second heart attacks, the FDA would not approve it, claiming defects in the study. Nonetheless, many doctors, albeit illegally, are prescribing the drug to heart-attack patients, convinced that it is beneficial. In fact, sales of the drug keep climbing, in this country and overseas. The laboratory which has manufactured the drug turned over the original study to an impartial review board and has begun to test the drug in England, Italy and South Africa.

Timothy E., fifty-five, who has had two heart attacks, plans to investigate both of these drugs, as well as the calcium-blocking agents.

Timothy's history is peppered with cardiac incidents, and he has angina, for which bypass surgery was recommended. But Timothy falls into the category of patients which has refused to undergo surgery. He is on a medical regimen and feels he is doing well.

It started in 1974 when Timothy, who is an artist, felt dizzy and clammy while at work in his newspaper office. He continued to feel uncomfortable although he did not have severe chest pain, but his doctor gave him electrocardiogram and enzyme tests that revealed he had indeed suffered a heart attack. However, he recuperated without complications.

At the time, Timothy says he was an "uninformed consumer." He had always been healthy, so he had never developed the habit of asking his doctor too many questions. He did not know what his cholesterol level was or how high his triglycerides were or even what his blood count was. "I only knew that I hadn't smoked for twelve years, and that was good," says Timothy. "But my doctor told me my blood work was normal. It never occurred to me to ask what that meant. Now I ask. What may be good enough for the doctor may not be good enough for me."

About six weeks after the heart attack, Timothy walked six blocks to his doctor's office. It was a lovely spring day, and he was accustomed to walking. But about halfway there, he felt discomfort—not pain—in his chest. He stopped to rest, and it disappeared. His physician told him it was probably angina and prescribed nitroglycerin tablets to place under his tongue.

"It helped me a lot," remembers Timothy. "I noticed that I could walk about five blocks before the pain started. Then I would put a nitro under my tongue and it disappeared rapidly."

Timothy's condition remained stable for about three months, but then the chest discomfort came more often. He could walk fewer and fewer blocks without stopping for relief from the little white tablet.

His second heart attack came without warning, while he was resting, watching television. This time, nitroglycerin didn't help the pain, and he was taken to the hospital in an ambulance. His attack was described as a mild one, and he remained in the hospital for only ten days.

But afterward, his doctor ordered a stress test. Timothy did poorly. Early in the test he experienced chest pain, and there were changes on the electrocardiogram being taken as he was exercising on the treadmill.

A catheterization soon afterward revealed that Timothy had three blockages: his right coronary artery was almost completely occluded; his circumflex was 80 percent blocked; and his left anterior descending artery was 70 percent clogged. There were no blockages, however, in the critical left main coronary artery. His physician told him that considerable collateral circulation had built up on his right coronary artery, which meant that the blood was reaching his heart through alternative channels which had been created by nature to compensate for the almost total blockage.

His cardiologist strongly recommended a heart-bypass operation, telling Timothy that he was a good candidate for the surgery.

But Timothy refused. "I wanted to try whatever noninvasive things I could first," he says. He had read somewhere about a glucose-tolerance test to check on low blood sugar, a condition known as *hypoglycemia*. "I had read that that could affect your whole system, and I wanted to see if I had it. My doctor didn't think it was necessary, but he went along."

Timothy did not have low blood sugar, but the test did show that his triglyceride level was 350, much too high. By this time, Timothy had begun delving into the medical books and was convinced that nutrition had a major role in heart disease.

His next step took him to a nationally known nutritionist, Dr. Willard Krehl, at Philadelphia's Thomas Jefferson University Medical Center. Dr. Krehl immediately put him on a 1,000-calorie-a-day diet. "It was tough to follow," Timothy says, "because I felt as though I were starving. But in six weeks, I had lost twenty-six pounds. My triglycerides had come down to one fifty-five, and my cholesterol level dropped from two seventy-five to two fourteen."

Timothy's cardiologist prescribed Inderal (40 mg. four times daily), a beta-blocker, to be used in conjunction with nitroglycerin. And Timothy continued in a vigorous self-help program which consisted of attention to diet and exercise. He walked two miles a day, barred sugar from his diet, took vitamins.

At one point, he tried to cut down his dose of Inderal (after checking with his doctor) because he felt it fatigued him and slowed him down. "It's almost like taking a tranquilizer," he says. But his heart rate increased a little, and his cardiologist advised him to resume the higher dose.

Today, Timothy feels as though he is in excellent health. His heart attacks seem like dim memories. But he continues to pore through medical journals. And he insists on knowing details about his medical condition. "It used to be, for instance," says Timothy, "that the doctor's nurse would call me on the telephone to read the results of my blood tests. She wouldn't give me numbers. She would just say, 'Potassium is normal; choles- terol level is normal.' Well, now I want to know what normal is. Is my potassium three point five, which is low- normal; or is it four point five, which is high-normal? Is my cholesterol one ninety or two seventy, all of which is in normal range? I want to be an active participant in my own health care."

Today, Timothy's cardiologist, the same cardiologist who encouraged him to undergo a bypass operation four years ago, is saying that he doesn't feel it is necessary. He is satisfied with Timothy's progress on medication and his altered life-style. But he insists on watching him closely for any changes that might warrant a different approach to his heart problems.

While no one denies that a patient's coronary anatomy (the extent and location of blocked arteries) is critical in determining how well he or she will do on either medical therapy or surgery, more doctors are feeling that personal attitudes and feelings count heavily toward the patient's well-being.

Philadelphia's Dr. Katz describes a patient who recov- ered well from bypass surgery. The patient, a fifty-two- year-old man, called him one Thanksgiving Day com- plaining of angina pain at rest. The patient was hospitalized, but the angina subsided quickly and he was released from the hospital. There were no problems until the following year, about four days before Thanksgiving, when the same thing occurred. "We talked about it," says Dr. Katz, "and we both realized that Thanksgiving time and November were difficult periods for this patient. His father had had a coronary in November. His father had died the following November. The patient himself had had a catheterization in November, and his bypass sur- gery had been done in November. He was experiencing what we call 'the anniversary reaction.' "

It has happened that a husband and wife develop angina and die in the same year. Or that a woman will have a heart attack soon after her husband. Or that a patient will have angina walking to the doctor's office, but not walking away from it. "The incidence of this sort of thing is much higher than you would expect," says Dr. Katz. "This is not technological data, but it cannot be overlooked as a prime factor in the history of angina."

When a person with angina, who has been doing well on a medical regimen, begins to have pain at rest, it is often a key signal that the condition is worsening. Some doctors will hospitalize the patient in an effort to control the pain. Nitroglycerin may be given intravenously to dilate the arteries and take the load off the heart. If that does not work, sometimes a device called an *intraaortic balloon pump* helps reduce the heart's load and enables it to work less. The device is inserted through an artery in the leg; the procedure is considered a relatively simple one, often done at bedside.

One of the difficulties in determining how well or how poorly medically treated patients do is that all medical treatment is not uniform. One patient may be receiving propranolol and another being maintained on nifedipine. Dosages vary from patient to patient. Life-style—including smoking habits, amount of exercise, diet—can be dramatically different from person to person. And the natural-history studies of persons with angina (their course without surgical intervention) were recorded at a time when beta-blockers and the newer calcium antagonists were not used.

Nonetheless, there have been many attempts to determine the prognosis for patients who are treated medically compared with those who undergo surgery (see Appendix 1).

A seven-year study at Duke University Medical Center looked at 1,214 medically treated patients with coronary disease to determine:

· how many of them suffered nonfatal heart attacks within seven years;
· how many of them died within seven years;
· which risk factors figured most heavily in producing heart attack or death.

The group studied was comprised of patients who had been catheterized at Duke between November 1969 and January 1978, and who had coronary disease of 75 percent or more in one or more major arteries.

The medical therapy of all patients included advice about modification of diet and other risk factors (such as smoking) and the use of short-acting nitrates, long-acting nitrates and beta-blocking agents.

Among these 1,214 patients, there were, in seven years, 245 deaths related to cardiac causes and 14 that were nonrelated. One hundred thirty-three patients (of whom 28 later died) experienced nonfatal heart attacks.

Persons with progressive chest pain were at greater risk. For instance, at five years, 48 percent of patients with this kind of pain experienced a heart attack or died. But only 29 percent of patients without progressive chest pain had similar experiences. The effect of progressive chest pain was the same in patients with one-, two- or three-vessel disease.

The study, which appeared in *Circulation*, pointed out that ventricular function, a potent predictor of survival, does not seem to influence who has or does not have a heart attack. And since having had a heart attack worsens the prognosis for a patient, the study's author says that "improving the long-term survival rate in patients with multivessel disease may depend on decreasing the incidence of nonfatal ischemic events [heart attacks]."

Conclusions are that:

- The natural history of coronary artery disease is a series of cardiac events.
- The number of blocked arteries, the extent to which they are blocked and the impairment of ventricular function are important determinants of the frequency of cardiac events.
- Progressive chest pain and Prinzmetal's angina (angina caused by spasm) are important predictors of a cardiac event, perhaps because the types of pain patterns represented by these two conditions indicate a critical shortage of oxygen to the heart.
- The probability of surviving a heart attack is strongly influenced by the quality of left ventricular function and the presence of disease of the left main coronary artery.
- Over a longer period of time, the extent of the diseased arteries and the progression of chest pain are probably the most important predictors of survival because they are related to the incidence of heart attack.

Dr. Harold Rutenberg, of Pennsylvania Hospital, emphasizes that "it is difficult to evaluate surgical treatment against medical treatment of patients because surgery is a standard, definitive procedure, while medical treatment varies among physicians.

"If patients are not receiving the optimal medical treatment for their conditions, they may not compare as favorably, especially where symptoms are concerned, against surgical patients as they would if they were on an aggressive medical regimen."

7 LIFE AFTER SURGERY

Joe L.'s problems began in August 1980, when he felt a strange sharp pain along the side of his neck. At first, he attributed it to recent dental work, but soon his mouth stopped hurting, while the pain in his neck persisted. Three days later, his neck hurt so much that he could hardly walk halfway around the metals-product shop where he was a production supervisor. At five-thirty in the morning, when he was ready to leave work, the pain came again, this time so jolting it almost took Joe's breath away.

The next day, Joe's doctor told him he had had a heart attack and hospitalized him for nine days. "He couldn't understand why I hadn't had even more pain than I described," says Joe, who is fifty-one, "but I have a good tolerance to pain, and he thinks I may have just suppressed it."

A month after Joe's release from the hospital, he enrolled in a cardiovascular rehabilitation program at Philadelphia's Albert Einstein Medical Center's Daroff Division. It is a regimen which involves attention to the "whole person" after heart surgery or a heart attack. There is meticulously prescribed exercise tailored to the needs of each person, education about the function of the

194

heart and modification of abuses to it, and help with psychological and social problems.

"What we do with each person depends on his or her condition and the goals each wants to attain," says Barbara Gleeson, who directs the program. "We don't believe in the philosophy that we have all the answers and that we keep patients in the dark. We want them to be educated enough to ask questions and to know more about how to help themselves."

Joe came to the program three times a week. He exercised on a treadmill, rode a stationary bicycle and learned how to keep his cholesterol level down. But three months later, he was given a stress test and was told that there was trouble with his heart. At the time, Joe's cholesterol level was 300, too high, but his blood pressure was normal. His parents, while they lived into their seventies, had both died as a result of heart disease.

A catheterization showed that there were four blockages, including two in the left anterior descending artery and one in the right coronary artery. Joe also had an *aneurysm* (a scarred area of the heart that can hold a lot of blood).

"I guess I'm a little unusual," Joe says. "When the doctor told me I needed surgery, I wasn't afraid. I just wanted to have it right away and have it over with. The doctor explained everything to my satisfaction, and I had confidence.

"I was afraid only one time," confesses Joe. "I was scheduled for surgery late in the afternoon, and my wife and children were there. But at three o'clock, they said they wouldn't be doing my operation that day because there was an emergency. I would have to wait until the next day.

"My family went to the cafeteria to get something to eat and then they were going home," says Joe. "But right after they left, the nurse came into my room, saying that plans had changed and they could take me that day after all.

"Well, I was really scared. My wife and children weren't there, and I felt so alone. I said, 'No, thank you. Tomorrow will be fine.'"

Joe's operation, in spite of the aneurysm which often increases the risk of surgery, went smoothly. Joe doesn't remember any pain. Even the tube in the throat, which most patients find the most uncomfortable part of the procedure, was gone before he was fully awake. "The only painful part was trying to cough," he says.

Joe moved quickly out of the intensive-care unit and would have gone home a few days later except for a slight infection that manifested itself by an elevated temperature. But it cleared quickly, and Joe was discharged.

On his way home from the hospital, he stopped at the familiar cardiovascular rehabilitation program to visit Ms. Gleeson and his other friends. "I wanted them to know I was OK and that I would be coming back as soon as my doctor would let me," Joe says.

Joe's doctor let him come back a month later. Joe's goals are to stay on a low-sodium diet to keep his blood pressure down, to keep his weight down (he dropped from 188 to 176 and wants to lose 11 more pounds) and reduce his cholesterol level (it has already dropped from 300 to 215).

"I have a positive attitude," says Joe. "My doctor says that if all patients had my attitude, many of them would have fewer problems after surgery."

It is true. A positive attitude makes a difference. There is a growing belief that personality, relationships with others, compliance with programs that will modify risk factors and employment status may be critical indications of who will do well after heart surgery or even after medical treatment for heart disease.

A study of thirty bypass patients at the University of North Carolina showed that, despite good physical results of the operation, 83 percent of patients were not employed and 57 percent were sexually impotent one to two years later. Some practiced a limited life-style, and there was a problem with low self-esteem, prolonged depression and distorted body image. The research results, which were published in the *American Journal of Psychiatry,* concluded that more attention must be paid to the psychological and social adjustment of bypass patients after surgery.

Researchers at Duke University, taking a cue from orthopedic surgeons who have long used psychological tests to determine which patients are likely to receive relief from low-back pain after surgery, have developed a similar process to study patients with coronary artery disease. Prospectively, the researchers looked at 538 patients who were treated medically for their coronary artery disease and 265 patients who had bypass surgery. The 546 men and 257 women were between 18 and 84 at the time of the study (1979).

After each patient had received angiography which confirmed the presence of blocked arteries, he or she was given a test to reveal the tendency toward hysteria and hypochrondria (heightened awareness of bodily functions and dependence on others).

Another questionnaire was designed to assess the person's perception of his place in society; in personal relationships with his family and friends; in his job, hobbies and patterns of exercise. The Duke scientists also noted whether the person had worked before treatment (medical or surgical) and whether he was employed afterward.

Six months later, 70 physical characteristics (including data from the electrocardiogram, results of catheterization, medical history) were evaluated, as were seventy psychosocial values. These 140 characteristics—the physical and psychosocial—were looked at as predictors of who would have reduced pain from angina after treatment.

Dr. Redford B. Williams, Jr., professor of psychiatry and associate professor of medicine at Duke, says, "Only three bits of data emerged as independent predictors of pain relief—hysteria level score, hypochondriasis-level score and employment status."

A normal hysteria level is less than 70, and the study showed marked relief of pain in 80 percent of the men and women in the study with hysteria scores less than 70, who were treated medically. When their hysteria level rose to 85 or more, only 40 percent obtained relief from angina. Persons with tendency toward hypochondria showed approximately the same thing. Lower hysteria and hypochondriasis scores were also associated with higher pain relief in the group of patients who received surgery.

Seventy percent of the men and women who were working and treated medically were free of pain, compared to 43 percent who were without pain in the group that was not employed. However, when treated by surgery, no significant differences in pain relief were evident in the working and nonworking group.

The study is continuing for several years to see whether the initial results continue.

The staffs at medical centers and hospitals where a lot of heart surgery is performed are aware that "peace of mind" can go a long way toward a patient's speedy recovery and ultimate quality of life. Therefore, they set up programs, prepare literature, give lectures and work with heart patients and their families to put them at ease before and after surgery. "We find it makes it easier if patients and their families know what to expect," says Chris Crumlish, a critical-care clinical specialist who used to work at Philadelphia's Lankenau Hospital. "That way they know that what they are experiencing is normal, and the families know, for instance, that nothing is wrong when they see all of those tubes and bottles. We think it makes a difference in the hospital, immediately after the operation, and when they get home. It is a shock for the family if they are not prepared."

The American Heart Association publishes a booklet called "Coronary Artery Bypass Graft Surgery," which explains not only the operation, but describes what will happen in the hospital immediately following surgery. Patients who have read the booklet say that the information it contains is reassuring and that, without having had it in advance, they would have experienced serious mental anguish.

It helped, for instance, to know that:

· There is a place where family members can wait during the surgery and that the surgeon will communicate with them as soon as the operation has been completed.

· After the surgery, all patients are sent to an intensive-care unit, where they remain for a day or a few days until they are moved to their rooms.

· Relatives are able to visit patients briefly while they are in the intensive-care unit. In fact, in most medical centers and hospitals, they can visit within an hour or two after the operation while the patient is still asleep.

· There will be many tubes and wires that are routinely attached to parts of the body during surgery and which will remain for varying lengths of time. The most uncomfortable will probably be the breathing tube, which is removed when breathing assistance is no longer required. This usually occurs within twenty-four hours after the operation.

- Patients in the intensive-care unit, because it is a twenty-four-hour beehive of activity, sometimes feel confused or disoriented. This temporary confusion usually resolves in a few days.
- It is normal to run a fever after the surgery, and the fever may last for a few days. Sometimes the patient will perspire heavily. It does not mean that anything is wrong.
- As soon as the breathing tube is removed, liquids can be given. Soft foods are soon added, and as soon as it can be tolerated, solid food may be eaten.
- To reduce the chance of pneumonia, it is important to do deep-breathing exercises and to cough. The nurses in the intensive-care unit will help by pounding patients on the back or against the sides of the chest.
- When patients return to their rooms, they will be doing some exercise right away. At first, it may be just sitting in a chair. The next day, it may be walking around the room or down the hall. Longer walks will help prepare patients to go home.
- Sponge baths are given right away, and in a few days, showers and shampoos are permissible.
- There is not usually severe pain, but medication is available to relieve discomfort.
- The incisions in the chest and leg (or legs) will begin to dry as they are exposed to the air. They can be washed with mild soap and water within a few days, and lotion may be applied later.
- The incision will gradually change in color from purple to red to pink and, eventually, will return to normal. Many people say they can hardly find their incisions once they have healed completely and returned to normal color.
- Most people stay in the hospital for seven to fourteen days and, if they live within driving distance, can go

home by automobile. If they must use other transportation—plane, train or bus—arrangements can be made to board in advance of other passengers.

The Cleveland Clinic has undertaken an intriguing experiment that seems to offer psychological and physical benefits to many patients. Patients who have stable coronary artery disease, but who need surgery, receive their laboratory tests and chest X rays as an out-patient on the night before surgery. The patient spends the night before the operation at home or in a hotel (if the patient is from out of town) with his or her family. The morning of the surgery, the patient walks to the hospital, is taken to a special part of the hospital where he or she is prepared for the operation. During this time, the family remains with him.

"Invariably, these patients are discharged about seven days after surgery," says Dr. Loop. "The savings in hospital charges amounts to about 11 percent of the total bill, and our patients say that they thoroughly enjoy spending the night before surgery with their families. I operate on five or six patients a week who come into the hospital under this plan."

The normal recovery period from heart-bypass surgery is from four to six weeks, during which time patients gradually return to their normal activities. It is important, in the beginning, not to become overtired or to set unrealistic goals. Many people feel more comfortable if they avoid big, heavy meals; eating smaller portions and more frequently is often more relaxing and can help an overweight person shed extra pounds.

Because it takes at least a month for the breastbone to heal completely, most physicians urge patients not to drive during that time. Riding in a car is all right, but not for extended periods of time at first. Lifting, moving furniture, vacuuming the rug or shoveling snow should not be resumed until checking with the doctor.

"The first month at home was the worst time for me," says Jim P., a robust man in his late forties. "I felt fine, but there was so much I wasn't allowed to do. No lifting, no pushing, no raking leaves. I tried reading, but how much can a guy read? All they let me do was walk. But my wife was working, so I decided to do little things at home. I would start dinner and set the table, dust the furniture, clean some drawers. I tried to keep myself as busy as I could until I went back to work." Jim, who is manager of a drugstore, returned to his job two months after his operation.

"Even now [eight months later], I am still numb around the incision, and my incision is still a little red," he says. "When the weather changes, I know it. My incision begins to pull and sting. But if it gets too uncomfortable, I use a heating pad. And basically, I feel pretty good."

Jim says that when he first came home from the hospital, he needed to rest at least twice a day, for about forty-five minutes each time. Other people find this unnecessary. Milwaukee's Dr. Dudley Johnson remembers a man who was out on the golf course twenty days after surgery.

After the first visit to the doctor (usually in four to six weeks), many men and women find they are able to resume activities such as tennis, swimming, horseback riding or jogging.

"Fortunately, I didn't have to wait that long to resume sex," says Mindy R., a pleasant, outgoing woman in her early fifties. Mindy had been married only three months to her second husband when she learned that she had blocked coronary arteries and opted for surgery. "I guess that what you worry about the most depends on which stage of life you're in," Mindy says. "Here I was, newly married, with a husband eight years younger than I, and sex was important. It was the second thing I asked my doctor about. The first thing was, 'What are my chances of surviving the operation?' I remember that the doctor said to me, 'Well, there's no question what your priorities are—life, then sex. You're going to do just fine.' "

Most people worry about what their sex lives will be like after the operation. Will sexual activity strain their hearts? Will it affect the incision? Will it induce a heart attack?

Physicians generally advise patients not to worry too much about sex. If they can relax and enjoy it without being overanxious, there is no reason why they can't begin having sex as soon as they feel ready. However, if they are tired, tense and troubled by it, it might be better to wait until they feel more comfortable.

Certain positions in sex may have to be avoided for a while if they are too uncomfortable. For instance, Mindy says that the traditional missionary position was impossible for her to tolerate in the weeks after surgery. "But actually, it was great," she says. "We became adventurous and discovered new ways. We never went back to the old style, even when I was able to."

A study on sex for heart patients, conducted by Dr. Herman Hellerstein, a Cleveland physician, reported that a person who has suffered a heart attack need not worry about sexual intercourse precipitating another heart attack. If a person can comfortably climb one or two flights of stairs, take a fast-paced walk, he should be able to have sex without anxiety, beginning, for most people, about six weeks after the heart attack.

There are exceptions, however. Extramarital sex may be more dangerous because of the guilt that often accompanies such activity, and sex in a marriage where there is a large age difference between the spouses may carry more risk.

Some patients need to take medications, such as beta-blockers or anticoagulants, even after surgery. Others say they have not touched a pill since the operation was performed. It depends on the patient—how free of pain he or she is after surgery, what the condition of the heart muscle is, whether there are any arrhythmias that need attention, if there was a history of heart attack before surgery, whether the patient is diabetic or hypertensive. Patients should ask their physicians the purpose of the medication prescribed if they do not understand its use.

"I thought that after surgery I would be able to stop my medicine for high blood pressure," says Henrietta T., fifty-two, who had a triple bypass operation in 1976. "I figured I would just throw away the bottle. So I was surprised when my doctor told me that my high blood pressure was not cured. I'm still taking diuretics and potassium supplements and some other things, too, all for blood pressure. I was disappointed that I couldn't stop taking them, but I realize it's important, and I don't miss a day."

Henrietta is correct. The way a person takes care of himself or herself after surgery is critical to survival and to the quality of life. Because atherosclerosis is a progressive disease, surgery cannot cure it. It can only slow it down. It is up to each person to do whatever possible to keep the condition from accelerating. The person who returns to a life of stress, smoking and soufflés runs a greater risk of continued problems than one who lives a more prudent life-style. Some people are disciplined and can make the appropriate changes in the way they live on their own. However, there is a growing realization that enrollment in a cardiac rehabilitation program, such as the one in Philadelphia, is the best way for many people to learn and maintain a healthy life-style.

"Our program is geared to people who have had any cardiac event [heart attack, severe angina] or who have had heart surgery," says Barbara Gleeson. "We offer no guarantees, but we feel hopeful that with good cardiac conditioning, they will do better."

Most people who enter the program do so three to six weeks after their heart attack or surgery, accompanied by full reports from their doctors which give details about their conditions.

The first step is a graded exercise test (a test that gradually increases the work load to determine a person's cardiovascular responses—blood pressure, heart rate). Then each person is asked to define his or her goals . . . physical, occupational and social. For some people, the goal is just general conditioning. For others, it is to strengthen a specific part of the body, such as leg or arm muscles. For others, the main goal is to be able to feel strong enough to return to work.

"Some of our patients come here years after an infarct [heart attack], and they are literally cardiac cripples," says Ms. Gleeson. "They have been at home, doing next to nothing. These people may not be able to go back to work after so long a time, or they may be past retirement age. But they can learn to do things around the house, some home repairs, maybe. They also learn to check their own heart rate, and if they get too tired, they can slow down or rest."

In any case, the results of the exercise test and the patient's goals are translated into a daily exercise prescription, one that is followed at the program (where patients usually come three times a week) and at home.

"We want to pay attention to the total person, not just his heart," says Ms. Gleeson. "So our program has three facets—the physical, educational and psychosocial support."

Ms. Gleeson wants her patients to be educated. She wants them to know how the heart functions, what their risk factors are, what the purpose of their medication is, which foods they should eat, how to check their own heart rate, how to judge appropriate levels of activity. She publishes newsletters, promotes discussion groups and invites family participation.

She stresses that prevention begins in childhood, so those enrolled in her program are encouraged to bring their children and grandchildren. "We want people to understand that it is their bodies, and they are entitled to know how to take care of themselves," she says. There are regular family nights with speakers who discuss such topics as nutrition, exercise, mental attitudes and adjustment to a chronic disease.

"Some people come to the program feeling depressed and anxious. The support they get from others who have been through similar experiences and are going through the same emotions helps a lot."

"The best part of coming here is getting to talk to everyone else," says Tom B., a fifty-five-year-old man who recently had heart-bypass surgery. "You think you feel bad, but then you see other people who also had heart surgery, and you can talk about it. If you get a pain, you think it is something terrible happening, but here you find that others have had the same pain at that stage after surgery, and you feel reassured that there isn't something wrong with you."

For patients who have been accustomed to being active and outgoing, the program provides an outlet until they can resume their normal schedule. Ms. Gleeson says it is especially beneficial to Type A personalities—those accustomed to working intensely and accomplishing a lot. "This gives them something to do and to work for. And that's very important at that stage of recovery."

Ms. Gleeson finds that people who are reached early and given the appropriate support and education are less likely to need psychotherapy later.

The exercise program at the center includes calisthenics, stretching and limbering exercises, followed by work on the treadmill, stationary bicycles or arm ergometers (machines which strengthen arm muscles). Patients learn to take their own pulse rate, and blood-pressure readings are taken before and after exercise. Ms. Gleeson says patients need conditioning exercise twenty to thirty minutes three times a week.

Attention to nutrition is a critical part of the rehabilitation program, and the recommended diet is one suggested by the American Heart Association. It limits intake of foods rich in cholesterol and saturated fats (such as butter); dramatically reduces the use of salt; and advocates baking, broiling and roasting of food instead of frying it.

Nutrition, in fact, is considered by many experts to be the key to improved well-being after surgery. Despite the debate about the influence of cholesterol on heart disease, the most weighty evidence strongly suggests that it is prudent for everyone, and especially those with heart disease, to limit the intake of cholesterol.

A number of extensive studies, including one of approximately 21,000 people in fifteen countries, correlated the severity of atherosclerosis found at autopsy with dietary habits of the populations. The populations which consumed more cholesterol and saturated fats had the most severe levels of atherosclerosis. Another research project called "The Seven Countries Study," which compared dietary habits among men in different areas of the world —including northern, eastern and southern Europe; the United States; and Japan—also found a strong relationship between the intake of saturated fats, the level of cholesterol found in the blood and the incidence of coronary artery disease. And an intriguing study of Japanese living in Japan, Hawaii and San Francisco showed that the incidence of coronary artery disease was lowest in Japan, where consumption of cholesterol is least; higher in Hawaii; and highest in San Francisco, where cholesterol and saturated fats comprise a heavy percentage of the diet.

The American Heart Association is recommending its diet for everyone, not only those afflicted by heart disease. It feels that it is safe, even for children, although it is still studying the ramifications of such a program on young people.

In fact, there is a growing feeling that cholesterol levels should be controlled beginning in childhood. Dr. Gerald Berenson of Louisiana State University found that some children as young as two already had cholesterol levels as high as young adults. By the time a child is eight, many researchers feel that cholesterol levels should be known, especially if heart disease runs in the family.

Unfortunately, many of the foods which form the basis of children's diets—hot dogs, for instance—are loaded with cholesterol or saturated fats. So are ice cream, cookies and store-bought cakes (they are high in saturated fats because those fats preserve the cakes longer).

The habits learned while young persist, and the adults who are addicted to pastries, butter and eggs are usually the ones who were nurtured on those foods. No matter. It is important, say many experts, to change those habits or, at least, to modify them. Often, this involves a new style of preparing food and will impose unpopular restrictions on other members of the family. At first, it may even create tensions because it may be felt that the needs of one family member are changing longtime, comfortable eating patterns for everyone.

However, many families are astonished at how easily they can become accustomed to—even enjoy—a new style of eating, especially when it is accompanied by an improved sense of well-being.

"If someone had told me I would eat potatoes without butter or actually prefer a banana to a piece of strawberry shortcake, I would have told them they were hallucinating," says Meryl V., whose husband had bypass surgery five years ago. "I thought I would prepare the foods he was supposed to have for him, but I would continue eating what I liked.

"But after a little while, I got tired of making two dinners. He would have fish, and I would have roast beef. I would steam his vegetables and sauté mine. It got to be too much work, too many pots. He couldn't eat my way, so I decided to eat his way.

"In a month I lost eight pounds, and I really felt better. Soon I stopped pouring salt on my food, and I was eating more fish than meat. And now I don't think I could go back to the other way."

The American Heart Association is promoting nutrition for healthy hearts and has begun working through the school system to reach children at an age when eating habits can be more easily modified. Its nutrition committee publishes literature, produces films and arranges media conferences to get its message across to the public.

Its current message is:

- Fat calories should comprise no more than 30–35 percent of total calories consumed (the average American consumes 40 percent of his or her diet in fats).
- Saturated-fat calories (butter, meat) should not exceed 10 percent of total calories.
- Carbohydrates, especially complex carbohydrates (starches), should replace the reduction in fat calories.
- Cholesterol intake should not exceed 300 milligrams a day.
- Total calorie intake should be reduced, if necessary, to achieve a desirable weight.

No one knows exactly how diets high in cholesterol and fats work to coat the coronary arteries with plaque, and it has even been suggested by some that reduced intake of fats and cholesterol will not be effective because the body produces its own cholesterol.

"It is true that the body produces its own cholesterol," says Dr. W. Virgil Brown, professor of medicine at Mt. Sinai School of Medicine in New York. "But cholesterol produced by the body does not usually push it up to the danger levels. It is the diet that does that. There is no question that you can reduce blood cholesterol through diet."

Another researcher, Dr. Robert W. Mahley, director of the Gladstone Foundation Laboratories for Cardiovascular Disease at the University of California in San Francisco, has found a mechanism through which diets high in fats and cholesterol can clog the coronary arteries. Cholesterol and other fats are carried in the blood stream in large protein molecules called lipoproteins. Dr. Mahley and his coinvestigators have discovered that a certain type of lipoprotein, called beta-very-low-density lipoprotein (beta-VLDL) delivers large quantities of cholesterol to cells from the artery wall in laboratory cultures. The cells, called macrophages, become foamy and fat-laden. Diet enters the picture because high intake of fats and cholesterol causes production of beta-VLDL in both man and animals. Beta-VLDL normally is not found when fat and cholesterol intake is low.

While it is generally accepted that high cholesterol and increased risk of heart disease go together, there has been some question about the relationship of low cholesterol levels and increased incidence of cancer, specifically colon cancer. Many people, confused by the conflicting reports they read, wonder if by changing their diets, they may not be substituting the risk of one disease for another.

Indeed, several studies correlate low cholesterol levels and cancer. Three (two reported in the British literature and one in America) suggested that higher cancer mortality may be associated with lower levels of blood cholesterol. Low cholesterol levels are usually those below 190.

However, other studies did not support these findings. And the position of the American Heart Association is that a "moderate dietary change to lower blood cholesterol is prudent. The incidence of coronary heart disease in our society remains very high, and this seems to be due to a significant extent to the high mean cholesterol in the U.S. public. Since the relation between high cholesterol and coronary heart disease is well established while that between low cholesterol and cancer is only tentative, an attempt to reduce coronary heart disease by cholesterol lowering seems justified."

The Heart Association concedes, however, that more investigation is needed to determine whether low cholesterol levels are, indeed, linked to some types of cancer.

Cholesterol is not the only fat in the blood, and it may not be the only culprit. High triglycerides (called hypertriglyceridemia) have also been linked to increased risk of heart disease, and there is no doubt that heart patients often have high triglycerides. But high triglycerides often coexist with other risk factors and may not, independently, be as responsible for heart disease as cholesterol levels. For instance, high triglyceride levels are usually associated with *reduced levels* of high-density lipoproteins (HDL—see Chapter 1), a condition associated with greater risk for coronary heart disease.

Because information so far is insufficient for a conclusive answer to the triglyceride riddle, it is felt by many experts that it is judicious for those who have had heart attacks or have undergone heart surgery to maintain normal triglyceride levels (this can be checked through simple blood tests). Triglycerides can be reduced in most people through lowering intake of simple carbohydrates and avoiding the use of alcohol.

What about the use of alcohol? Many people who have been through heart surgery wonder whether they should be drinking at all. Evidence about the influence of alcohol on heart disease is still inconclusive, but a few recent studies indicate that, contrary to expectations, consumption of alcohol may even be beneficial.

It is known that moderate to excessive use of alcohol leads to increased blood lipid levels, especially triglyceride levels, and that increased blood lipids are associated with a higher incidence of cardiovascular disease. Therefore, it has been expected that regular alcohol drinkers would tend to have a higher incidence of coronary artery disease. It does not seem to be so.

A study of 909 men in two Milwaukee hospitals over a four-year period showed that those who abstained from alcohol use or consumed moderate amounts of alcohol (less than one ounce a week) had more coronary artery disease than those who drank more.

This was especially remarkable since the patients with heavier alcohol consumption were also hypertensive, were heavy smokers and had higher levels of blood triglycerides (alcohol is known to increase blood triglyceride levels). The researchers feel that the most plausible explanation for the protective effect of alcohol is its association with increased levels of high-density lipoprotein (the "good" cholesterol).

There are other studies, however, which do not show a correlation between drinking and lowered incidence of coronary artery disease. And still others show an association between moderate consumption of beer, wine and liquor; increase in high-density lipoprotein (the "good" cholesterol); and less incidence of heart disease.

Therefore, the American Heart Association's Nutrition

Committee feels that alcohol taken in large amounts is toxic to the heart, may destroy heart muscle and contribute to atherosclerosis through its effect on blood fats in some people. The committee suggests the "prudent" use of alcohol.

Changes in diet alone, however, are less effective than adoption of a comprehensive program which includes lowering high blood pressure, eliminating cigarette smoking, controlling diabetes, limiting stress and getting more exercise.

Many people can control high blood pressure through changes in the way they eat. Eliminating salt is a major factor. Although the body needs less than one gram of salt a day, most people consume from eight to ten grams. This results in salt-loaded tissues which retain fluid and put extra strain on the heart. Cutting down on salt usually means eliminating processed foods which are rich in salt, cutting out such foods as soy sauce, pork, salted crackers, pretzels, potato chips, sausage and bacon.

Three studies, conducted by the United States Department of Agriculture, indicate that balancing the fat intake between saturated and unsaturated fats can also lower blood pressure. They examined seventy men and women between forty and sixty years of age who were healthy except for moderate elevations in their blood pressure. When their fat intake was balanced, their pressures became normal, in spite of the fact that their intake of salt was not reduced.

There is little dispute that cessation of smoking is essential for those afflicted with heart problems. The effects of nicotine and carbon monoxide have been shown to affect the transportation and use of oxygen in the body, the heart rate and the blood pressure. The risk of "sudden death" from heart attack is related to the number of cigarettes smoked a day.

The Framingham Study found that the heavy cigarette

smoker is subject to eight times the exposure of carbon monoxide allowable in industry. And it is felt that the death rate from heart disease among women may soon approach that of their male counterparts because of the increase in the numbers of women who smoke.

But the effect of cigarette smoking can be reversed, and there is a rapid beneficial effect to those who stop smoking. Those who have stopped smoking cigarettes have only half the risk of cardiac problems of those who continue to smoke. The benefits usually begin within a year after smoking has stopped. There is evidence, however, that the benefits of quitting smoking are not as great to the elderly as they are to the young. For both men and women, the effect of cigarette smoking on coronary heart disease diminishes with age. Overall mortality, however, is distinctly greater in both young and old cigarette smokers.

The benefits of exercise are supported by a number of studies, although it is generally felt that exercise, without attention to other risk factors of heart disease, will be of little benefit. One of the most important effects of regular exercise may be that it seems to raise the high-density lipoprotein level in the blood, which may have a protective quality against heart disease.

Exercise should be carefully monitored by a physician and should be engaged in regularly, at least three times a week, for twenty to thirty consecutive minutes. Exercise can be brisk (four to five miles per hour) walking (which some experts feel is the best activity), bicycling (ten to fourteen miles an hour), swimming, tennis, handball or active sports played vigorously.

Some research shows that men benefit more from exercise than women, perhaps because of a difference in the ability of females to metabolize cholesterol. Dr. Lloyd Laubach of the University of Dayton says that while exercise raises the level of the protective substance—high-density lipoproteins—in men, it does not do that for women.

"Exercise counts," says Dr. William Kannel, former director of the Framingham Study, "but not nearly as much as giving up smoking, lowering cholesterol or lowering blood pressure. If a person stops smoking, he can cut his risk of having a heart attack by fifty percent, and it would take a lot of running to achieve that."

While many people are able to take positive steps, such as changing their diets, exercising more and giving up smoking, it is often more difficult to reduce stress and convert from an "A-type" to a more placid personality.

Yet, many experts, including those who were skeptical at first, believe that this personality type may be as much a risk factor for heart disease as the more established ones, such as high blood pressure, smoking and high cholesterol levels.

A study underway at the National Heart, Lung, and Blood Institute of 900 heart-attack victims is examining the effects of modifying Type A behavior. So far, second heart attacks have occurred less frequently among the persons who have successfully changed their Type A behavior.

Preliminary results indicate that it may be even more important to reduce anger and hostility than to cut down on working hours, eliminate stressful activities and lessen the sense of urgency typical of Type A personalities.

"I know I should work less and spend more time with my family and not go crazy when I'm stuck in a long line at a bridge opening," says Spencer C., a forty-three-year-old accountant who has had a triple bypass operation. "But I can't help it. I'm just built that way. I have a hard time delegating responsibility. I feel as though if I don't do it, it won't get done right. Even when I'm on vacation,

I call my office twice a day and I bring work with me. I
get impatient reading a book, and I'm bored at movies.
Doing my job and doing it well is the most important
thing to me."

Spencer has a lot of company. Part of the current study
is to motivate such people to change their behavior. Since
all of the participants have suffered a heart attack, it is
hoped that they would be frightened enough to consider
behavior changes seriously. All of them have a videotaped
interview to determine their Type A score. Dr. Meyer
Friedman, who, with Dr. Ray H. Rosenman, popularized
Type A personalities in the late 1960s, says that more than
98 percent of persons who have had heart attacks have
high scores.

Techniques for altering frenzied behavior are suggested. For instance, if someone is stranded in a long line
of cars on the highway, he or she might be told to make
productive use of the time, instead of wasting energy on
anger. Listening to the radio is a possibility. Thinking
about something, such as vacation plans or the next day's
activities, is another possibility. Or if the delay is especially long and traffic is at a standstill, the time could be
filled by writing a letter, making a shopping list or planning a dinner party.

A Montreal psychologist, Dr. Ethyl Roskies, believes
that if Type A's can become convinced that their way of
life is unproductive and inefficient and that there is a
better way, it can be successful in producing change.

"I used to be your typical A personality," says Miriam
F., a forty-five-year-old journalist and broadcaster. "If
every minute of my time wasn't accounted for, I thought
I was a failure. I expected perfection, not only from myself
but from my husband and children. If they got B's on their
report cards, I was disturbed because they were not A's.
If my husband made a wrong turn on the highway, I

would be upset because we had wasted time going out of our way.

"Well, after my heart operation [Miriam had four by-passes because of intractable angina], my priorities changed. I realized that all of the things I had thought were so important were less important. Somehow, the work I had done before going to the hospital got done, in spite of my absence from my newspaper and my radio station.

"The laundry got done in spite of me, and the kids didn't look like vagrants. The house wasn't as spotless as it was when I was taking care of it, but it didn't matter. Nothing awful happened because I wasn't orchestrating every activity. And I actually felt a sense of relief that I didn't have to be perfect."

There are specific relaxation methods suggested by several researchers. The most popular, perhaps, are those of Dr. Herbert Benson of Harvard University. Dr. Benson believes that different things work for different people. For some, it may be meditation. For others, it may be religion. For some, it may be recreation. But he feels that learning to relax is important for everyone and certainly is critical for heart patients. Like cigarette smoking, stress, it is felt, lowers the level of the protective high-density lipoproteins (HDL) and has an adverse effect on the heart.

Miriam says that while she has learned to relax more, she was eager to get back to work and, in fact, was covering newspaper assignments within six weeks after her discharge from the hospital.

Is Miriam typical?

Because more than 75 percent of patients who were previously incapacitated by angina obtain partial or full relief of symptoms after surgery, it would be expected that they would return to work and to productive activity afterward. They do not.

A study of 350 patients at the University of Alabama Medical Center showed no improvement in return to work or the number of hours worked a year after bypass surgery. Of 132 patients who did not work or worked only part-time before surgery, three-quarters continued in that status. Only 25 percent went back to full-time jobs.

Of 218 patients who had worked full-time before surgery, 66 percent continued at their jobs. The other 34 percent went back to part-time work or were not working at all.

Another research project, conducted by the Seattle Heart Watch, showed that 75 percent of 1,198 patients were working three months before bypass surgery, but only 62 percent was working full-time one year later. When these patients were compared to a group treated medically, there was no evidence that those who had surgery were more likely to return to work.

In both the surgical and medical groups, fewer patients continued working if they were over fifty-five years old, had twelve years or less of education, had not been working for three months or more before surgery (for the surgical group) or catheterization (for the medical group), or were suffering from severe and limiting angina before catheterization or surgery.

For both groups, the strongest predictor of who would return to work was the employment status before catheterization or surgery. Those patients who were employed full-time before catheterization or surgery were more likely to be employed a year later.

Age was the next most important predictor, followed by education, severity of angina before surgery or catheterization and the length of time the patient was unemployed before surgery or catheterization.

The study's authors concluded that, because coronary surgery does relieve symptoms and improve performance on exercise, the reasons for failure to return to work must be largely nonmedical. They suggest the patient's fears; economic incentives to retire (such as pension payments, Social Security benefits, disability insurance); and competition for jobs by younger, healthier people.

Other researchers suggest that some people do not return to work because they feel as though their jobs may have triggered their heart problems. And many people change occupations after their surgery to an area that is less stressful or less demanding physically. However, the study by the Seattle Heart Watch revealed little evidence of change in occupation.

In addition, many heart patients enjoy the attention lavished on them by friends and family and are reluctant to risk their loss by returning to work.

In a paper written by Drs. Albert Oberman and Nicholas T. Kouchoukos of the University of Alabama, it is stated that the family and even the physician may reinforce dependent behavior by overly protecting the patient. They cite a Canadian study which showed that physicians often advise patients to stay away from work and certify them as disabled, even though exercise capabilities are greater than necessary to perform the job.

But Sammy K., fifty-seven, who worked as a foreman for a clothing manufacturer before his triple bypass surgery, says he wanted to return to work, but his employer rejected him. "He was afraid I wouldn't be able to perform, and while I was out, I was replaced by someone younger who didn't have health problems," Sammy says. "They offered me early retirement and I took it, even though I would have preferred to go back on the job."

A Milwaukee study revealed that while some people retire and others return to their previous jobs, there is a sizable group that changes occupations—some to more sedentary work and some to more demanding work.

However, the decision to switch jobs had nothing to do with the person's age or with the presence of angina. It concludes that "the knowledge of having cardiac disease must have great impact on the work capabilities or desires in those whom it affects . . . whereas the severity of heart disease exerts a relatively minor effect upon whether an individual makes job changes."

Bypass surgery itself is expensive, from $10,000 to $15,000 for every operation performed. But even more expensive is the economic drain caused by the continued unemployment of those who have the operation. In fact, one of the justifications for bypass surgery has been the expectation that patients who have it can go from invalidism to productive employment. This expectation, however, has not been realized in many cases.

No matter how patients feel after surgery—whether depressed or exhilarated, suffering from continued angina or free of pain, back at work or vegetating at home—almost everyone says that they benefit most from the support they get from others who have had the surgery.

"It is impossible for someone who hasn't been through this to know what it is like," says Elaine E., an attractive woman in her mid-fifties who had the bypass operation in the early 1970s. "When I went in for it, no one I knew had ever heard of it, and I didn't know one person who had had it. There was nobody to ask a question of, nobody to tell me what I could expect or how I might feel later. My doctor did his best, but he never had the surgery, and there were certain questions he couldn't answer and certain feelings he had never felt."

Elaine was one of the relatively small number of people who had a terrifying experience in the intensive-care unit after surgery. "I remember it well," she says. "There is no sense of time. The room is unisex—men and women sleeping next to each other. There are nurses milling

around all the time. Monitors beep all the time. Two people died while I was there, and one had to be resuscitated.
I didn't know where I was. And every time I looked toward the nurses' station, I kept seeing a circle of witches
dancing around a boiling pot. I know now that they
weren't there, but I can still see them, and it has been ten
years."

Because Elaine remembers how isolated she felt, she
became active in Philadelphia's Zipper Club, an organiza-
tion comprised of men and women who have had heart
surgery. The club publishes a newsletter, arranges peri-
odic meetings where a facet of heart surgery is discussed
and, most important, provides comfort and support to
members and to new heart-surgery candidates.

"I talk to people several times a week, people who are
thinking about the surgery," says Elaine. "I tell them everything that happened to me so they have a better idea
of what to expect. Not that every person is the same," she
concedes. "But we have lots of people that someone can
talk to, and it means everything. I wish I had had it. But
since I didn't, I want to help other people who are in the
same boat. . . ."

The Zipper Club, which was founded in Pennsylvania
in 1974, has chapters in several states. Its members work
with hospitals which often encourage their visits to patients prior to surgery. Whenever possible, the Zipper
Club will try to match the patient with a member who is
the same age and has a similar medical problem.

Two days before his operation (a quadruple bypass), Ed
P. was visited by a Zipper Club member, two years
younger than Ed who is almost fifty-three, who had had
similar surgery three years earlier. Both men had had no
history of heart attack, and their heart muscle (ventricular
function) had been normal.

"That visit meant more to me than anything," Ed says.

"I felt I could ask questions and tell him how I felt more than I could with anyone else. I wanted to know how he felt right after the surgery, when he went back to work, when he could have sex again, how much pain there was. I worried about the incision in the leg because I'm a tennis player, and I wasn't sure I'd be able to play again."

After Ed's operation, his Zipper Club companion visited him again, and they have remained good friends. "It is a shared experience, a bond that we have in common," Ed says. "Now we help each other."

The spouses of heart-bypass patients say that they, too, derive comfort and help from other wives and husbands. Consider Connie M., who says that her husband's heart surgery threw her into a panic. "I was fine before the surgery because there was a clear path to follow," she said. "He was going to go to the hospital. He would have the operation. I would visit him. He was in the hands of a superb doctor. Then he would come home, and all would be well."

According to Connie, all was not well. "I didn't know how fragile he was, really," says Connie, "so I didn't know how to act. If I got angry about something, I was afraid to show it because I thought it might upset him. If I wanted to go somewhere, I was afraid to suggest it because he might be tired. If I was interested in sex and he made no move, I was hesitant to bring it up because it might not be good for him.

"It affected our relations with the children. I wouldn't let them do anything out of line because I was afraid of how it would affect Lou," Connie says. "If they didn't hang up their coats, I would yell at them because I thought Lou would lose his temper if he saw their stuff around. I made them keep the stereo down and lower their voices. I walked on eggshells because I was so terrified.

"It wasn't until I met other wives that I realized that

what I was going through wasn't unique . . . that everyone has those same feelings and reactions. Other women told me how they handled those problems. One special woman, who has since become one of my good friends, explained that I had a right to live comfortably, too, that I didn't have to be as cautious as I had been, that my husband was not as fragile as I thought. Without that support and encouragement, I'm not sure our marriage or I could have survived."

Carol T., a fifty-two-year-old woman, says that her husband's disposition was not the problem. It was his memory loss and his inability to express himself well that were most traumatic. "Here was a man who was a nationally recognized courtroom attorney," says Carol. "He had been so glib and so articulate . . . now he was groping for words. He would tell me, 'I know the word I want, but I can't find it.' He was so frustrated he would pound on the wall until he cried.

"Not remembering our next-door neighbor's name was no fun either," says Carol. "It was painful to see. But a friend whose husband had had a similar experience after his bypass assured me that it was transient."

Now, three years later, Carol's husband has regained many of his lost skills. "But I'm afraid he will never be quite the same," Carol says. "And I still have the need to talk about it with other wives of bypass patients. I don't know why, but it makes me feel less alone."

Anna D. had other problems after her husband returned home after surgery. "He was hostile, angry all the time," she says. "Nothing I did was right. He made me feel so guilty, as though it was I who had caused his heart problems. I was his target, the one he yelled at, the one he blamed. He was obnoxious. Then I would look at his incision and remember all he had been through and feel guilty for hating him."

Anna went to a psychiatrist without her husband's

knowledge, because she felt she could no longer tolerate her life. She was thinking seriously of divorce. But contact with the wife of a friend who had undergone the surgery convinced her to stick it out a little longer.

"His wife, Lila, told me that a lot of men go through that stage. You are there, and you're the one they take their problems out on. She said it happened to her husband, too, but that in about six months, his disposition returned to normal."

It took a little longer for Anna's husband to become his cheery self again; more than a year, in fact. But she says that sharing her misery and anxiety made all the difference and, indeed, saved her marriage.

8 ARE THERE ALTERNATIVES TO SURGERY?

Frank M. has not had an easy life. While he was in his twenties, he was diagnosed as having a progressive retina disease, and by the time he was forty-five, he was totally blind.

When he was thirty-nine, and while he still had some sight, he experienced a heart attack from which it took him a year to return to his normal life-style.

"For one year after my heart attack, I took it easy and did next to nothing," Frank remembers. "Then I returned to the mainstream of living and went back to work." Frank and his wife operated a retail seafood business. "For another year, I watched myself, but then I began to get angina. I always felt fatigued and short of breath. If I lifted anything or did anything stressful, I got the pain."

As time went on, Frank's condition worsened. He swallowed dozens of pills, including Inderal, Isordil and Coumadin, an anticoagulant. There was a period of time when he was taking 320 mg. of Inderal a day.

"Nothing helped me," Frank says. "I was never able to go back to a full day's work, and I always felt lousy. I was physically and emotionally spent. Every medication I took had some side effect. It was a seventeen-year-long nightmare."

In 1978, Frank and his wife went to California for six months. When they returned, Frank was sicker than he had ever been. He could barely walk. He couldn't even get through a morning shower without tiring. "I had a bell in the shower, and I had to ring for my wife halfway through my shower so she could help me get washed," he recalls. "Then she would help me to bed. I was in awful shape."

Frank's cardiologist told him he had to have an angiogram, probably followed by bypass surgery.

"I figured he knew what he was talking about, so I did what many people do . . . I let my doctor be responsible for my life," says Frank.

Frank's catheterization showed three blockages, one of 85 percent, one of 65 percent and one of 70 percent. Surgery was strongly urged.

"I remember that the night before surgery, I was lying in my bed in the hospital, frightened, and I began to cry," says Frank. "A young nurse walked in and looked at me and ran out to call someone. A few minutes later, a large, big-bosomed nurse came in, sat on the side of my bed and cradled me in her arms. She spoke to me in a soothing, loving voice and told me that I was in good hands and everything was going to be OK. It was sort of like getting back to the womb. I decided I was going to give my body to the surgeons. I lay back and said, 'I'm no longer responsible for my body. I am putting myself in very capable hands, and everything will be OK.'"

Frank says that it wasn't OK at all. After his surgery (which was supposed to be a triple bypass but was only a double because one artery was not graftable), he developed pericarditis, a painful inflammation of the membrane which surrounds the heart. And he still had angina.

Thirty days after surgery, he felt no better. His cardiologist, whom he calls a "sweet, gentle, competent man," assured him that he would improve. Ninety days later, he had a stress test, and it was found that his exercise capacity was worse than it had been before surgery.

"It was disappointing," says Frank. "And three months later when another stress test had even worse results, I went into a state of anger, anxiety and depression. I was falling to pieces . . . that's what happens when you let your head go.

"My doctor told me that what they did to me mechanically [in the bypass operation] had to work," Frank says. "If I was still having trouble, it was in my head, and I needed to see a psychiatrist. I left his office and told my wife that I was going to get a second opinion.

"The cardiologist I consulted told me he wanted to take another angiogram and see whether I could be helped further surgically. I said nothing but took my wife and headed for the nearest restaurant. I ordered eggs and bacon and corn muffins dripping with butter and fudge cake with ice cream. Everything I knew was bad for me. And I told my wife I wasn't going to have my body invaded again. I said I would become a cardiac cripple."

A few months later, Frank heard a television show which described a program in California which seemed to be helping people with heart problems. It was a program that combined diet and exercise and, according to the television report, was achieving near miracles with very sick people.

"I wasn't too thrilled at first, because I was a two-martini, bottle-of-wine, cherries-jubilee man," says Frank. "But I'm also an eight-cylinder man, and I was running on one cylinder and I wasn't happy about it. So I decided to learn more about this program and begin to follow it."

Frank says he began to see results in ten days. "I couldn't believe it," he says. "I hadn't been able to walk ten feet, and now I could walk around the block. In a few more days, I could walk three blocks, then four blocks, then five or six. Then I took walks in the park with my dog [Frank has a seeing-eye dog]. One day by accident I walked up a hill and found myself running down. I felt euphoric that I could do this. And I started jogging, turned from a cardiac cripple to a whole person. But I was still afraid that it wouldn't last."

Frank's fears were unfounded. He continued to improve, his angina vanished and he asked his doctor to modify his medication. Gradually, he reduced his intake of drugs, and since 1979, Frank has needed no medication.

"If someone asked me today, Should I have open-heart surgery? I would tell them to give this program a thirty-day trial first."

The program that Frank says is responsible for his well-being is the Pritikin program, a diet and exercise regimen dramatically different from that followed by the average American. The diet is low in cholesterol, which Nathan Pritikin says blocks the arteries; low in fats, which he claims could block circulation; and low in protein, which he says could create a negative mineral balance. It is high in complex carbohydrates, because they maintain the appropriate blood-sugar balance; and high in fiber, which Pritikin says has a beneficial effect.

Nathan Pritikin is not a doctor, and he does not mind admitting that he has "no credentials." In fact, he is a college dropout who has been studying the human body for forty years. His background is in electronics, chemistry and physics. About twenty years ago, Pritikin himself experienced heart problems and put himself on a low-fat, low-cholesterol diet, which he says cured him. His cholesterol level dropped from 300 to 100. Today he advocates the diet for the treatment of a variety of disorders, including diabetes, hypertension and coronary artery disease.

The key, Pritikin claims, is the level of cholesterol in the body. This level, he says, closely correlates with the incidence of heart disease. In this country, a cholesterol level of 160 to 300 has been considered normal (although the American Heart Association prefers cholesterol levels that hover around 200 or less). But Pritikin insists that deaths from heart disease strike people with "normal" cholesterol levels. "Persons with cholesterol levels of two hundred sixty or more have a five hundred percent greater chance of succumbing to heart disease," he says.

Pritikin urges everyone to find out what his or her cholesterol levels are and encourages reducing them to no more than 160.

Eliminating fats is crucial. The average American diet has a 40 percent fat content, and each year most people consume approximately 150 pounds of fat, the saturated part of which escalates the cholesterol count, which contributes to coronary artery disease. Pritikin claims his diet reduces cholesterol by 10 percent in six days and by 25 percent in four weeks.

Forbidden foods on the Pritikin diet usually include oils, sugars, fatty meats, organ meats, shrimp, egg yolks, dairy products (except non-fat), nuts (except chestnuts), jams and jellies, fruits or fruit juices with added sugar, commercial breads and cereals, alcohol, coffee, tea, cola, salt and white rice. Poultry, fish and lean beef is limited to one-and-a-half pounds a week.

If that sounds as though there is nothing left to eat, Pritikin assures that there are still plenty of "goodies" to choose from, and that once a person has tried his diet, chances are that he or she will stick with it. The rewards, according to Pritikin, are freedom from the ravages of debilitating degenerative diseases and a longer, healthier life during which people feel younger, look better and are more energetic. The promise of relative immunity from heart disease may be the diet's greatest attraction.

Consider Jack L., a sixty-year-old periodontist who has suffered with angina since 1961. Although his discomfort has grown through the years, he did not want to undergo a catheterization and bypass surgery.

"My internist has always been conservative about surgery, but when I finally saw a cardiologist in 1977 because my angina was worse, he thought I should go for an angiogram," Jack says. "But I hemmed and hawed, trying to make up my mind about it, and I delayed long enough that in the interim, I read an article about this guy in California who was helping people like me through diet and exercise.

"I asked my cardiologist about it, and he said, with no enthusiasm, that I could try it if I wanted to. But later, when he realized I was serious about going out to Santa Barbara, he called my wife and told her he thought I was nuts."

It has been almost five years since then, and Jack does not think he is nuts at all. In fact, he is convinced that the Pritikin program has helped him. And he says that if he could adhere to it strictly, he would feel even better.

Before Jack tried the Pritikin program, he was complaining of angina attacks which came frequently, several times a week. He was taking nitroglycerin when the pain came and Inderal every day. His son lives in a house located on a hill, and Jack found it a chore to visit. "I had to take at least three nitros every time I climbed that hill," he remembers. "I had little energy, and even though I kept up my practice, I was tired a lot and couldn't move as quickly as I liked.

"I've always figured that if I could have medicine instead of surgery, I would prefer it. And carrying that concept further, I figured if I could use diet rather than medicine, I would like that even better. I knew I would consider surgery if I really had to. But if there was an alternative, I'd want to try it."

Jack tried the Pritikin program in mid-1977. At the time, his blood pressure was normal, but his cholesterol was 275. "My cardiologist told me that wasn't too bad," says Jack, "but Pritikin thought it was a disaster."

Jack spent a month in Santa Barbara where Nathan Pritikin operates a Longevity Center. He ate meals different from those to which he was accustomed, and he walked four to five miles a day.

When he came home, he had lost weight and his cholesterol level had dropped to 160. Since that time, it has slowly crept up to a high of 210, but it has never approached the 275 of his pre-Pritikin days.

"Now I walk up that hill to my son's house without needing to take a nitro," Jack says. "But I have to admit that I still get angina, and it is just as frequent, perhaps more frequent than it used to be. But I know I'm not adhering strictly to the Pritikin program. I only walk about a mile a day, and I cheat on the diet. If I kept it up, I know I would feel better. . . . That Pritikin, I think he knows what he's talking about. . . ."

Many medical doctors agree that Pritikin's program can lead the way to a healthy heart. Philadelphia's Dr. Gerald Lemole, who has performed hundreds of heart operations, has his family on a modified version of the diet. Dr. Lemole's breakfast every day includes a bowl of oatmeal with four teaspoons of bran and one-half teaspoon of fructose, a natural sweetener. His lunch consists of a glass of vegetable juice, celery and carrot sticks, and a salad. Dinner always includes soup, salad, perhaps a vegetable platter or a bowl of brown rice with chicken or a plate of whole-wheat spaghetti with an oil-free tomato sauce.

Cleveland's Dr. Floyd Loop says, "I'm not a nutritionist,

but I think that Pritikin has the best low-cholesterol diet and program that there is. Pritikin goes very far when he says that he can regress some coronary artery disease; but for a good rehabilitative effort, I think it's probably very beneficial."

And while the American Heart Association's diet seems almost like a banquet compared to Pritikin's restricted regimen, many of the same principles—low cholesterol, low fat, more complex carbohydrates—exist in both. Dr. W. Virgil Brown, professor of medicine at Mt. Sinai School of Medicine in New York, says that there is a problem with credibility when you are talking about a program such as Pritikin's, where the successes are documented only by testimonial evidence (rather than scientific tests). And he does feel that the Pritikin diet is unnecessarily restrictive. But he admits that "we could probably wipe out coronary artery disease if we followed it."

Other physicians agree that the basic concept of the Pritikin program makes sense. No one can argue with a plan that helps a person shed extra pounds, encourages exercise and lowers cholesterol. But there is considerable dispute about whether blocked arteries will become un-blocked. And because the diet is so unpalatable to so many people, some physicians suggest that it be practiced in moderation.

Pritikin responds, "Would you take poison in moderation?"

Still other physicians object to the "antiphysician" attitude that they say the Pritikin program promotes. "I worry about patients who turn away from doctors because they think Pritikin has cured them, then run into problems later—and they do—and don't know where to turn," says Philadelphia's Dr. Richard Helfant.

Meanwhile, Pritikin's program seems to be gaining in popularity, and there are dozens of anecdotal stories of patients whose angina has improved or vanished after a month of Pritikin-style living.

The Pritikin Research Foundation, which is studying the causes and treatment of degenerative diseases, conducted a five-year follow-up of sixty-four patients who attended the Longevity Center. All of them had documented coronary artery disease and had been recommended for coronary artery bypass surgery. The follow-up was done by telephone.

Of the sixty-four patients, eleven had undergone bypass surgery, one had died of cancer of the bladder and one had died of "sudden death," presumably caused by cardiac problems. One had died while running and one died during surgery for a valve replacement. Eighty-five percent of the patients said they had a 50 percent or higher compliance to the Pritikin program, and 54 percent said they were walking six or more miles a week. The report concludes that the 0.6 percent annual cardiac-related mortality rate is lower than that reported by other groups for either medical or surgical patients.

Another project, called "Regression of Atherosclerosis Through Diet and Exercise," conducted in cooperation with the Department of Surgery at the UCLA School of Medicine, reported on three cases of "significant regression of atherosclerosis through diet and exercise."

One of them is a fifty-three-year-old contractor who began a running program in September 1978 and developed chest pain which radiated to his arms. A treadmill test, however, showed normal results with the patient performing to maximum capacity. But the pain continued almost daily and was eventually coming two to three times every day.

An angiogram was performed at the Texas Heart Institute in November 1978 which showed three obstructions. The left anterior descending artery had a 90 percent blockage, and the other two blockages were in medium-sized arteries. It was therefore decided to begin the patient on medical therapy.

At the time, the patient's cholesterol level was 275, and his triglycerides were 153. He weighed 182.

On his own, the contractor decided to modify his diet and reduce his cholesterol through the Pritikin program. After following the program independently for several weeks, he decided to enter the Longevity Center in January 1979. By that time, his angina attacks had already decreased in number.

At the end of his stay at the program, he was running six miles and walking four miles a day. He was no longer taking Inderal. At discharge, his two stress tests were normal, and his cholesterol level had been reduced to 133. His triglycerides were lowered to 121.

In the fall of 1980, a second angiogram, also done at the Texas Heart Institute, showed significant regression in two of his three diseased vessels. The blockage in the left anterior descending artery was reduced from 90 percent to 40–50 percent.

Pritikin says, "It is too late to discredit me. There are too many cases to demonstrate the improvements . . . only a foolish or unmotivated person would voluntarily abandon the program's enormous rewards."

He agrees that more research is needed to document the results of adherence to his program. But he says that "in the meantime, it does seem to have halted progress of coronary artery disease in numerous cases, and adherence is just a matter of education."

Loring C., a forty-three-year-old pilot who lives in Connecticut, had his first chest pain in October 1978. It occurred within a half-hour after awakening in the morning, for no apparent reason and without precipitation. "I wasn't running or exercising when it happened," Loring remembers. "In fact, I was drinking a cup of leftover coffee from the night before, so I thought I was having indigestion." But when the pain grew more intense and spread to his left shoulder, Loring decided to check in at the emergency room of the nearest hospital.

"They took an electrocardiogram and blood samples to check my enzymes, and treated me as though I had had a heart attack," Loring remembers. However, after two days in the intensive-care unit, the consensus was that there had been no heart attack. Perhaps he had had an angina attack.

One of the staff doctors was curious because the pain had lasted almost a half-hour, longer than would be expected if it were angina, and he began to ask Loring questions about his history. As he thought back, Loring remembered that the previous summer, after a big meal and while playing softball, he had had a minor episode with the same kind of sensation. Loring was sent for a stress test, which was normal. Then he was advised to have a heart catheterization. "I didn't know much about a catheterization, but I figured if the doctors said I needed it, I probably did," Loring remembers.

The catheterization revealed three blockages: one of 70 percent in the left anterior descending artery; another of 90 percent in a minor distal artery; and a smaller blockage —40–60 percent—in a branch artery. "They [the doctors] led me to believe that I was in serious trouble, and they immediately recommended a bypass operation," Loring says.

But Loring was hesitant. He knew that heart surgery would disqualify him from flying. He felt well, having only slight angina on extreme exertion, and he was not certain that he wanted or needed an operation.

"On the other hand, I was afraid if I didn't have it, I

might have a heart attack," Loring remembers. "So I decided to think it over for a few weeks."

Loring finally decided that he ought to have the operation. He consulted a surgeon in Hartford, whom he
remembers as being "very casual" about the surgery. "He
told me it was no big deal, that he did lots of these things
on Navy pilots and the Navy let them fly. . . . He made it
sound routine, but I was thinking—they split you from
head to waist, stop your heart, give it a thump and hope
it starts again . . . I almost had a heart attack just talking
about it," says Loring.

"Even as I made the decision, I was having second
thoughts about it. I began doing a lot of reading, and I
found that while the operation was often successful initially, sometimes patients had to go back for second or
third operations. I wasn't too happy about the prospect."

Despite his misgivings, Loring arranged to have his surgery done one Monday morning in December 1978. The
night before, he saw an article in the magazine section of
his local paper, which described a procedure called *angioplasty,* which could sometimes be used as an alternative
to bypass surgery. The next day, Loring contacted the
office of Dr. Simon H. Stertzer at Lenox Hill Hospital in
New York and explained his situation to the doctor's sec-
retary. After talking with Dr. Stertzer, she told him to
bring the films from his catheterization and come to New
York Wednesday morning.

"I canceled my surgery, telling them that I wanted a
second opinion," Loring says, "and I went to the hospital
and demanded my films [from the catheterization]. They
didn't want to give them to me, but I insisted."

In New York, Loring says Dr. Stertzer gave him a different picture. "He said that the distal artery that I was so
concerned about because it was ninety percent blocked
wasn't strategic and that it would probably not be bypass-

able, anyway," Loring remembers. "He told me that I might have trouble eventually, but that my situation wasn't critical enough to warrant bypass surgery at that moment. He also said that he thought the technique he was using could help me."

The technique used by Dr. Stertzer is called Percutaneous Transluminal Coronary Angioplasty, or simply PTCA or angioplasty. It was first used in the coronary arteries in 1977 at the Zurich Medical College in Switzerland by Dr. Andreas Grüntzig, who was influenced by the 1964 work of Dr. Charles T. Dotter and Dr. Melvin P. Judkins, radiologists at the University of Oregon Medical School. These men had successfully opened up narrowed leg and pelvic arteries to compress the blockages. The first person on whom they used the technique was an eighty-three-year-old woman with gangrene, for whom amputation of her foot had been suggested. She refused to have the procedure, saying that she would "rather die with both feet on," and was referred to Dr. Dotter. It took twenty minutes to dilate the narrowed area, and the woman's pain in the affected foot quickly subsided. She had had three irreversibly gangrenous toes which sloughed spontaneously when she began to walk again for the first time in six months, and she remained ambulatory until she died of heart failure three years later—with both feet on.

Dr. Grüntzig, using a modification of the Dotter technique, developed an alternative therapy to bypass surgery for certain kinds of coronary artery blockages. (Dr. Grüntzig is now at Emory University.)

The procedure, following the same principle as catheterization, involves snaking a catheter through an arm or leg artery into the affected coronary artery. When the tip of the catheter reaches the spot where the artery is blocked, a tiny sausage-shaped balloon is inflated with a hydraulically powered inflation device and compresses the blockage so it becomes smaller and thus increases the diameter of the vessel, permitting blood to flow through freely. Even a small increase in the radius of an artery can result in a noticeable increase in the flow of blood.

An angiogram is usually taken right before and right after the procedure. Even if there has been a previous catheterization, there is often a delay of weeks or months before the patient undergoes PTCA. During that time, the occlusions may have increased to the point where they totally block the arteries, or other developments may contraindicate the efficacy of PTCA. The follow-up angiogram will assess results of the procedure.

PTCA, if it can be used, has many advantages over surgery. There is no chest incision, and the trauma of an operation, a ten-day hospital stay and a convalescence of a month to six weeks can be avoided. The procedure usually takes about two hours and can be done in the cardiac catheterization laboratory. Patients leave the hospital in a day or two and can often return to work within a week.

However, not everyone is a candidate for PTCA. Persons on whom it is most effective are those who have had symptoms for less than a year, which would indicate that the lesions are not too old or too hard and are more likely to respond to compression.

It is better if the blockages are located near the origin of the vessel, are not too long and are symmetrical (not all on one side of the vessel wall). The patients should have serious angina that has not responded to medical treatment.

It is felt that approximately 10 percent of those who have coronary artery disease would meet these criteria. By 1980, 1,500 cases were done in this country.

Most patients who have the procedure have only single-vessel disease, although there have been cases where persons with double- or triple-vessel disease have been successfully treated.

"It is safest to use the procedure on single-vessel disease," explains Dr. Lamberto G. Bentivoglio, clinical professor of medicine at the Medical College of Pennsylvania, "because if the blocked vessel is damaged during the procedure serious complications are less likely."

However, Dr. Bentivoglio says that a few skilled practitioners who have been doing PTCA for a number of years are having some success with two- and even three-vessel disease, and can sometimes perform PTCA on vessels that have already been bypassed through surgery. "This usage of the procedure should be limited to doctors with a high degree of expertise and is at present strictly investigational," he says.

Persons who undergo angioplasty must understand that the procedure may not work, and if complications arise, he or she must be prepared to undergo bypass surgery immediately. In all cases, it is essential to have a surgical team ready to operate in the event it becomes necessary.

And because the procedure is still relatively new, long-term results are not yet known. Dr. Bentivoglio says that there is about a 15 percent chance of recurrence of coronary blockage within six months in patients who are treated successfully. But these patients can often receive PTCA again, usually with good results.

Because of the excellent results achieved by Dr. Grüntzig and his colleagues in Switzerland (between 1977 and January 1979, they performed more than 50 PTCA procedures, with approximately 60 percent success), the National Heart, Lung, and Blood Institute, in the spring of 1979, began to evaluate the technique.

A voluntary registry was discussed at an international workshop on PTCA on the campus of the National Institutes of Health in June 1979. The workshop, organized by Dr. Michael Mock, then the chief of the cardiac diseases branch of the National Heart, Lung, and Blood Institute (now with the Mayo Clinic), developed guidelines for the operation of the registry. The concept for such a registry was enthusiastically supported by the cardiology community, and by February 19, 1981, 1,116 patients from 69 centers were enrolled.

The mean age of the registry patients was 51.6 years, and the mean duration of angina was four months. Most of the patients (78 percent) had single-vessel disease; 19.3 percent had double- or triple-vessel disease; and a small number, 2.4 percent, had left main disease. Most (76 percent) were male, and 46 percent were employed full-time when they were first evaluated.

Other characteristics were:

- Thirty-five percent were cigarette smokers, and another 36 percent were former smokers.
- Twenty-five percent had a history of cholesterol levels greater than 250.
- Eight percent had a history of diabetes.
- Twenty-eight percent had a history of hypertension.
- Thirty-two percent had family history of premature coronary artery disease.
- Twenty-five percent had a history of heart attack.
- Ninety-six percent of the patients had chest pain, with 29 percent having had symptoms less than one month.
- Twenty-seven percent of patients had a good ejection fraction—more than 70 percent. In 6 percent of patients, ejection fraction was less than 30 percent.

The artery on which most of the procedures were performed was the left anterior descending. Twenty-three percent of patients had angioplasty on the right coronary artery, and 5 percent in the circumflex artery. Two percent had blockages in the left main artery, and 3 percent had the procedure for blockages in a bypass graft (where there had been earlier bypass surgery).

In 5 percent of patients, angioplasty was attempted for multiple-vessel disease.

These were the results:

- Sixty-two percent of blockages were successfully treated (success was defined as a 20 percent or greater decrease in the blockage). The procedure was most effective in the left anterior descending (66 percent), and least effective (33 percent) in the circumflex artery.
- When the procedure was not effective, it was usually because the blockage was too tight. When a blockage, through which a catheter could be passed, could not be dilated, it was usually because the lesion was too rigid.
- There were 439 complications reported on 216 patients, including in-hospital heart attack in 4.4 percent; in-hospital death in 1.3 percent (0.7 percent in patients who had not had previous bypass surgery, and 8.1 percent in patients who had been bypassed earlier). Emergency bypass surgery was performed on 6.6 percent of patients during their initial hospitalization.

Three-quarters of the patients followed up needed no other therapeutic procedure.

"This method is certainly preferable to having an operation," says Charles O., a forty-five-year-old man who had had PTCA just twenty-four hours earlier.

"I work as a mechanic at an oil refinery," Charles says, "and I do a lot of lifting and heavy work. One day it was really weird. In the morning I felt fine. In the afternoon I began getting pain in my chest and shortness of breath. It happened again, on and off, for the next two days, and finally I went to the first-aid department. They called my family doctor, who sent me to a cardiologist at Crozier-

Chester Medical Center [in Delaware]. The electrocardiogram they gave me was normal, and they talked about giving me a stress test but felt it was too risky. So they gave me a catheterization, which showed that I had one blocked artery."

After consulting with other physicians, Charles was told that he was probably a candidate for PTCA, and he was referred to Dr. Bentivoglio in Philadelphia.

"The procedure was no problem," says Charles. "It took about two hours, and I was awake the whole time. Every so often, they asked me to cough, but that was about it. I felt fine right after it was done, and I feel fine now. I'm eating regularly, and I expect to go back to work next week. . . ."

Several investigators in the United States are enthusiastic about the results with PTCA. The first 220 attempted uses of the procedure by Dr. Simon H. Stertzer and his colleagues at New York's Lenox Hill Hospital Center resulted in a success rate of 64 percent and an 14.1 percent recurrence rate during a mean follow-up period of ten months. The success rate was highest when the blockage treated was located in the left anterior descending artery. Dr. Stertzer does not know whether the lower success rate with blockages in the right coronary artery reflects the age and inflexibility of the obstruction, or whether blockages in that area are merely harder to reach and break up. However, with experience, success with blockages in the right coronary artery is improving.

In Dr. Stertzer's group of 220 patients, there were eleven patients with left main disease, and ten of them were successfully treated with PTCA. However, two patients experienced recurrence during the follow-up period, which ranged from one week to ten months. One hundred four of one hundred forty-two blockages in the left anterior descending artery were dilated successfully, with nine recurrences during the follow-up period. When the left circumflex branch was involved, the success rate was six out of eleven. But when the obstruction was in the right coronary artery, only sixteen of thirty-four could be treated with success.

Dr. Grüntzig and his group at Emory University are treating up to five patients a day with PTCA. When the procedure is applied to patients with single-vessel disease, the success rate ranges from 88–95 percent. "It is a major step that we have brought this procedure to be routine," says Dr. Grüntzig. "You can only do this if you diminish the complication rate." Dr. Grüntzig says that a fair figure, one that should be readily approachable by centers experienced in PTCA, is a 90 percent success rate with a 3 percent complication rate, when dealing with single-vessel disease. When a patient is being treated for multiple-vessel disease (which is a newer application of PTCA), the success rate (because of the learning curve which must be experienced for any new use of a procedure) would be expected to be lower at first.

Dr. Gruntzig says that for PTCA he will accept a person with double-vessel disease if his arteries appear (on angiography) to be acceptable for dilatation.

There seems no question but that PTCA is effective on certain groups of patients and is a less invasive and less costly procedure than bypass surgery. (More than 110,000 bypass operations are performed each year at a cost of approximately $1 billion annually.) The risk of PTCA on patients with single-vessel disease and without prior bypass surgery is equivalent to that of patients undergoing bypass surgery. However, as Dr. Bentivoglio points out, "We are getting equivalent results, but we are comparing one procedure [PTCA] which is in its infancy with another [bypass surgery] which is in its maturity. Each of us who is doing PTCA has experienced a learning curve, and we are doing better all the time."

Dr. Stertzer is confident that in the future the technique will be used more aggressively in more classifications of patients. He has treated the largest numbers of patients with left main disease and says that the results are encouraging. However, he stresses that it (PTCA on left main lesion) is an investigative procedure, and no one should be doing it except those who have a lot of experience and who are evaluating it as a separate procedure (from that done on single-vessel disease).

It is expected that as PTCA becomes more refined, its risk for patients with single-vessel disease may drop even below that of bypass surgery. However, it is still regarded as an innovative approach, and only through skillfully conducted scientific studies and follow-up of patients will the value of the technique be more clearly defined.

Frank S., sixty-three, and Joe M., sixty, were relaxing in comfortable canvas lounge chairs placed side by side and facing each other. Frank, who has thick white hair, was wearing plaid Bermuda shorts, an orange shirt and orange socks with folded cuffs. His friend Joe was dressed in a white knit sport shirt and tan pants. The two men talked about their health, their families and the tragedy of the baseball strike. Every so often, Joe would munch on a peanut-butter cracker, and Frank would glance at the newspaper that was folded in his lap.

The men might have been on a beach in Florida or on the deck of a posh ocean liner. But they were not. They were spending several hours in a small room that is part of the Philadelphia offices of Dr. Lloyd Grumbles. Both men had bottles of a clear fluid dripping slowly into their bodies intravenously, and both said that the treatment they were receiving was painless.

The treatment is called *chelation therapy,* a highly controversial technique through which, say its practitioners, clogged coronary arteries can often be cleared. It is a technique that has been approved for use in this country only for the removal of heavy-metal poisoning, especially lead poisoning. But its advocates are suggesting it as a viable alternative to coronary artery surgery.

"Unfortunately, there were a couple of unscrupulous practitioners of chelation therapy, men who would chelate anybody for anything," says one of the country's leading advocates of the technique. "And they have given the treatment a bad name in local medical societies."

Others claim that the problem is purely economic and that it is the income that would be lost to practitioners of traditional medicine that keeps them from recognizing the benefits of chelation.

The medical establishment calls these claims nonsense. It scoffs at the technique, insists it is of no value to heart patients and suggests that it can even be dangerous. Furthermore, there have been no scientific studies to demonstrate that the treatment has any benefit at all.

"The whole thing is a bag of wind," says Dr. Marvin Murphy, senior author of the famous Veterans Administration study on coronary artery bypass surgery.

"There is not a shred of evidence that shows that this treatment does anybody with heart disease any good at all," says Philadelphia cardiologist Dr. Richard Helfant.

And the American Medical Association declares that there is no scientific evidence whatever that chelation therapy is effective for the treatment of atherosclerosis.

Nonetheless, some heart patients who have heard about the treatment are willing to try it instead of undergoing surgery.

Forty-one-year-old Mickey A., for instance, says, "I know there is no scientific evidence that this chelation therapy will help me. And I have even heard that a few people have died from it. But I have no symptoms of coronary artery disease [Mickey's stress test was abnormal, and a subsequent catheterization showed blockages in two arteries], and there is no scientific evidence that a bypass operation will prolong my life, either. And people die on the operating table, too. So in the face of two treatments, both without scientific evidence of prolonging my life, I'll take chelation over surgery."

"Chelate" comes from the Greek word *chele*, which refers to the claw of a crab or lobster; it implies the ability to "claw out" or "pull out" of the body certain harmful substances. Its approved use is for the removal of heavy-metal poisoning—lead, mercury, arsenic—from the body. "Chelation is the only way to get it out of the body," explains Pennsylvania Hospital's associate physician of medicine, Dr. Robert E. Gerhardt.

Chelation works this way: Small amounts of an amino acid, disodium ethylenediaminetetraacetic acid (EDTA), are injected intravenously into the body. EDTA may be sodium-based or calcium-based. It is the calcium-based EDTA that is used in lead poisoning. In these cases, the EDTA binds to the lead in the body in such a way that it becomes soluble and can be drawn out of the body through the urine. When the EDTA is sodium-based, says its users, it binds to the calcium in the tissues and draws it out through the kidneys and into the urine in the same way. It is the ability of EDTA to bind metal ions that is the basis of chelation therapy. When EDTA binds with calcium or other heavy metal, in effect, it latches on to it and carries it through the kidneys into the urine and out of the body.

The use of chelation therapy to remove calcium deposits from the human body was first described by Dr. Norman Clarke, former director of research at the Providence Hospital in Southfield, Michigan. However, an attempt to duplicate Dr. Clarke's results by Dr. J. Roderick Kitchell and his colleagues failed to see clinical improvement in patients after chelation therapy.

Furthermore, in later years when some of the patients died, there were autopsies performed on three of them, showing that two of the three still had calcified coronary arteries.

Critics of Dr. Kitchell's work say that he abandoned his project too soon because he did not observe immediate improvement, noting that it takes chelation therapy a while to work. And that a re-evaluation of the patients after three months revealed that nine of the ten showed improvement from angina.

In an article they wrote for *Osteopathic Annals,* Drs. Garry F. Gordon and Robert B. Vance point out that the autopsy results led to the "erroneous conclusion that the treatments were not clinically useful in coronary disease as the effects were not lasting. . . . But subsequent years have taught us much about the natural history of arteriosclerosis, and no one, including surgeons, expects to permanently alter the course of arteriosclerosis with a single-modality approach today." Dr. Gordon says that EDTA has the same effect as the calcium antagonists described in Chapter 6.

Dr. Norman Clarke, Jr., son of the man who first described chelation therapy in the medical literature, has prescribed this treatment since 1956. He does not think that it is a replacement for the coronary artery bypass operation and says that he often sends his patients for surgery when he feels they will benefit from it.

"When patients have left main coronary artery disease or have unstable angina, I feel that surgery is the route for them to take," says Dr. Clarke. "But where the vessels are too small to bypass, or the disease is too widespread, or the disease is stable, allowing time to treat it, or the patient doesn't want an operation, I feel chelation should be tried. It is not a cure-all, but neither is bypass surgery. Chelation does improve blood flow."

Dr. Clarke says he has had good results over the years

with many patients, as measured by improvement in their symptoms, better tolerance of exercise and fewer subsequent cardiovascular complications.

He objects to pitting coronary artery surgery against chelation therapy as a treatment for angina, and he does not approve of "chelation clinics," which are set up only to dispense chelation therapy. "I take care of people," he says, "and select the treatment that is appropriate for each person considering the overall health problems."

Unlike some practitioners, he does not try to change his patients' life-styles, nutritional habits or exercise patterns when he starts them on chelation therapy. "I believe in a nutritional program and in appropriate exercise, but not at first," says Dr. Clarke. "I don't want to confuse the issue by changing everything at once. If you change a lot of things and a patient improves, you don't know what it was that made him better."

Despite the claims of its advocates, there is no scientific evidence, no double-blind studies, to indicate the value of chelation therapy. There are just the anecdotal stories told by patients and practitioners, in which traditional medicine places no faith.

Consider for instance Donald P., a fifty-three-year-old man who had been interested in health foods and vitamin therapy for years because he had a son with learning disabilities, who, he says, had improved on a diet-vitamin regimen.

In the summer of 1978, Donald began to experience angina. The pain came suddenly and grew rapidly in severity. After a few weeks, he had angina even when he was resting or after eating a meal. Within two months, he couldn't even climb the stairs without being halted by wrenching pain in the chest.

Donald was given a thallium stress test which showed that he had a blockage in his arteries, and he was placed on medication—Inderal, Isordil and a nitrate ointment which he applied to his skin. He achieved only minimal relief, and his doctor wanted to schedule him for a heart catheterization and possible bypass operation.

However, while he was waiting for a catheterization date, his wife read an article about chelation therapy and urged him to look into it.

"I was a little skeptical," said Donald, "because the article said that it was a potent medication that had dangers and had to be administered carefully. It mentioned kidney damage, and I wasn't sure I wanted to get involved with it.

"Instead, I put myself on the Pritikin diet, and I followed it very strictly. I did not do the exercise because I didn't have the energy, but I observed the diet to the letter. No oil. No sugar. Nothing. I stayed on it for two months—my brother was on it, and it helped him—but it didn't help me. I was still in pain."

Donald decided to try chelation therapy. He consulted Dr. Harold Buttram, a general practitioner in Quakertown, Pennsylvania, who practices chelation therapy and has a reputation for being a conservative physician.

"I had sixteen chelation treatments, but after the tenth one, I could feel a significant improvement. I had very little pain, and by the time the treatments were over, I had stopped taking all of my medicine. I had no pain except for the times when I would be exercising in extremely cold weather."

The following year, Donald returned to Dr. Buttram for fifteen more chelation treatments. "After that, I felt really good," he says. "I continued with the diet, but not as strictly as I had been. At this point, I can exercise with no pain, and I can even jog and repair my car and feel good."

In addition to the chelation treatments, Donald takes minerals and vitamins—four grams of Vitamin C; 800

units of Vitamin E; magnesium; potassium; zinc; selenium; chromium; manganese; iron; and copper every day.

His diet is still severely restricted, and he eats almost no meat. But Donald says that strict adherence to the diet is the only way he can keep his cholesterol and triglyceride levels down. His cholesterol which, before changing his diet, was between 400 and 500 is now 190. And his triglyceride level which used to be 300 is now 80.

"I give credit to the chelation therapy and the diet," Donald says. "I would recommend them highly."

Quakertown's Dr. Buttram admits that chelation therapy can be dangerous but says it is rarely so if it is administered and monitored carefully. Fear of kidney failure is of the greatest concern because a lot of toxic material is being eliminated through the kidneys.

And because EDTA is not selective, it takes out the good with the bad. Not only will it remove toxic metals, it will also eliminate B vitamins, which Dr. Buttram says must be replaced, or the treatment will do more harm than good.

"There have been claims that chelation therapy is dangerous," says Dr. Clarke. "But it just isn't so if it is administered properly. I don't have significant side effects in my patients."

Practitioners of chelation therapy often perform hair analysis on their patients, which they say can determine mineral deficiencies, and blood tests to determine vitamin deficiencies. Oral supplements are given, as well as vitamin supplements, which are given intravenously along with the EDTA. Dr. Grumbles, for instance, combines 15 grams of vitamin C, along with magnesium, in the EDTA solution that he uses to chelate his patients.

While some practitioners insist that chelation therapy is the answer to clogged arteries, others, like Dr. Buttram, are more conservative. "My basic philosophy is that if there is a proven medical therapy that is effective for a condition, I recommend it," Dr. Buttram says. "Chelation therapy is still experimental. There are certain lesions [blockages] in the arteries where surgery is the treatment of choice. In those cases, the patient should have it. But in marginal situations [where it is not certain that surgery can help, or there is small-vessel disease], I think they have everything to gain by giving chelation a try."

Dr. Buttram says that he sees some patients whom he feels should consider surgery, but they don't want to have it. And there are others who would agree to have an operation, but whose coronary anatomy is not amenable to it. "In these cases, I'll chelate them, but it isn't usually very effective," he says.

It is essential that the person doing chelation therapy be thoroughly trained. Dr. Buttram says it is like brain surgery—it is a definite skill and takes training and experience to gain expertise. It is critical to know, for instance, who are *not* candidates for chelation therapy; persons with compromised kidney function, for instance, may be rejected.

And there is agreement among practitioners that chelation will not work unless the person receiving it makes an effort to alter his life-style. Dr. Buttram emphasizes the importance of a change in diet. He thinks chelation therapy in combination with the Pritikin program "brings great results."

Some practitioners say that twenty treatments relieve angina in 70 percent of patients, thirty treatments in 90 percent and forty treatments in 98 percent. The treatments cost about eighty-five to one hundred dollars each, depending on the practitioner, and many hospital-insurance plans will not pay for them; they are not considered part of the mainstream of medicine.

Nevertheless, patients are often willing to bear the expense themselves to avoid the operating table. Frank, for example, the man described earlier, says he would rather pay for the cost of chelation therapy than take the risk of undergoing an operation. "Besides, the doctors told me I couldn't have the operation, even if I wanted to. They said my disease was too widespread and my arteries weren't bypassable."

Frank had had a heart attack in 1958 but did not experience angina until 1976. Until that time, he played golf three times a week and operated a service station. Inderal and nitroglycerin did not help him, and when he was told he was not a candidate for surgery, he decided to try chelation therapy, which he had learned about from his brother-in-law. At the time Frank was interviewed, he had had twenty treatments, with no change in the way he felt.

Joe, the other patient described earlier, has had high blood pressure since he was seventeen and began to experience angina in 1972. Nitroglycerin tablets and Isordil helped him a little, but his angina grew progressively worse. "I could only walk one block and make only one-half of a flight of stairs before I got the pain," he says.

"My doctor wanted me to go for a catheterization and bypass surgery," Joe says. "But I didn't want to go for it. I belong to the Conservative Book Club and saw a book advertised about chelation therapy. I was quite interested, and I bought it. I checked with the Academy of Medical Preventics in California, and they gave me a couple of doctors' names in the East where I live. And here I am."

Joe has taken twelve chelation treatments and says he felt better even after the first one. He says he can walk up to a mile now and go upstairs without pain. When he does get the pain, however, it is the same as it was before—still intense and still incapacitating.

Dr. Buttram believes that it is "bureaucracy, money and lack of vision" that is keeping chelation therapy from getting a fair test on the market. He says it would take millions of dollars to conduct the kind of study that would result in approval of chelation therapy—or any new drug —by the Food and Drug Administration. Pharmaceutical companies are not interested because the drug used in chelation therapy has been in use since the 1920s, and it cannot be patented. Therefore, no drug company is willing to make the investment."

The medical establishment argues that it is not economics that keeps chelation therapy from approval as a treatment for angina. They say it is simply a lack of scientifically sound evidence that it is effective.

"If you study the history of science, every new thing goes through a phase where there has been establishment reaction to it," says Dr. Buttram. "If we only had the vision . . ."

Fifty-one-year-old Peter R. had a heart attack in 1977. Since that time, he has suffered moderate angina whenever he exerts himself or is under stress. Peter's cholesterol level is 281 (too high), but his blood pressure is normal at 110/80. A catherization of his heart showed that Peter has three-vessel coronary artery disease with 40 percent blockages in his left anterior descending coronary artery, circumflex artery and right coronary artery.

In January 1981, Peter underwent bypass surgery at Philadelphia's Lankenau Hospital, but it was not his coronary arteries that were bypassed. He received a *partial ileal bypass,* a relatively simple operation that has the effect of reducing the amount of cholesterol that circulates through the blood.

The operation works this way. An incision, about five inches in length, is made in the lower right quadrant of the abdomen, and the ilium—a lower section of the small intestine—is bypassed by severing it and attaching it to a portion of the large intestine. The portion bypassed is closed off, but the blood supply remains intact so that the tissue stays alive and the segment remains connected to the intestinal tract.

This process reroutes cholesterol-containing materials (bile acids and salts) as well as cholesterol itself so that they do not go into the liver, which ordinarily recirculates them throughout the body but now, sends them to the colon, where they are lost in the stool. In this manner, the body can reduce its blood cholesterol level by 40 percent or more.

The operation has no side effects, except that those who have had it have a tendency toward diarrhea (patients usually have two to three bowel movements a day after the surgery), and the body's ability to absorb vitamin B-12 is compromised. Most patients' bowel habits become almost normal as time passes, and the vitamin B-12 deficiency is counteracted through injections of the vitamin four or six times a year. The effects of the surgery are lasting, with most patients sustaining the lower cholesterol level; however, the surgery is reversible at any time, if the patient desires.

(It is not the same operation as the much-publicized jejuno-ileal bypass that some people have undergone to achieve weight reduction, and the two should not be confused.)

The operation is not a new one, and there is no question that it lowers a person's cholesterol level. The riddle is: Will lowering cholesterol reduce the development of atherosclerosis and its complications?

Within a few years, the answer should be known. If it is affirmative, it is felt by some that the partial ileal bypass could possibly replace the coronary artery bypass operation for significant numbers of patients and be used as a preventive measure for countless others.

Atherosclerosis is not a new disease. There is evidence that Egyptian mummies embalmed between 1580 B.C. and 525 A.D. had it. And the mirror writings of Leonardo da Vinci show that he was the first person to describe and draw the deposits of atherosclerosis and to suggest that sudden death might be caused by thickening of the blood vessels leading to the heart.

Since the early 1900s, evidence has been accumulating that points the finger at cholesterol as the culprit in the development of atherosclerosis. Still, there is controversy about whether reducing cholesterol will indeed have an effect on coronary artery disease.

Peter is one of approximately 1,000 men and women in this country who will help us find out. He is participating in a five-year-study funded by the National Heart, Lung, and Blood Institute, which will prove once and for all whether lower cholesterol is or is not correlated to the stabilization—or even regression—of atherosclerosis.

The National Institutes of Health considers it a critical study, commenting, "It is the one study most likely to provide direct evidence . . . of the efficacy of reducing cardiovascular risk of life-threatening ischemic episodes [heart attack, sudden death, angina, etc.] in high-risk individuals [those with high cholesterol levels] who are already affected with advanced atherosclerosis."

"There is so much money being spent on treating the final complications of one disease [atherosclerosis]," says Dr. Henry S. Sawin, Co-Principal Investigator of the study at the Lankenau Medical Research Center. "But atherosclerosis is a progressive disease . . . this effort is designed to see if the disease itself can be treated."

The study is known as POSCH (Program on the Surgical Control of the Hyperlipidemias). *Hyperlipidemia* is the

term for the condition of having high levels of fat—cholesterol and/or triglycerides—in the blood. The centers
conducting the study are: the Medical Schools of the University of Minnesota (where the surgery originated), University of Arkansas, University of Southern California and
Philadelphia's Lankenau Medical Research Center.

In the mid 1960s, Dr. Henry Buchwald and his colleagues at the University of Minnesota publis'ed their
first experiments, which showed that bypassing the portion of the small intestine responsible for absorbing and
recirculating cholesterol resulted in a 28 percent reduction of blood cholesterol in white New Zealand rabbits.
The animals lived a normal life span following the surgery, with no weight loss or nutritional deficiencies. The
findings were duplicated and confirmed in another variety of rabbit, in pigs, dogs and rhesus monkeys.

The first such operation on a human, specifically to reduce cholesterol circulating in the blood, was performed
on May 29, 1963. Several hundred patients have been
operated on since, and the operation has become a standard procedure to manage hyperlipidemia. However, its
acceptance has been slow because the effect of lowering
cholesterol on the atherosclerotic process has been open
to question and because there is a natural tendency to
avoid surgical procedures when possible.

However, the average reduction in cholesterol among
those who have had the surgery, a reduction sustained
without the use of medication, is an incredible 40 percent.
This is considerably more than has been achieved through
changes in diet or through ingestion of drugs such as clofibrate, cholestyramine or nicotinic acid, the most traditional lipid-lowering medications.

Cholesterol that is reduced through diet cannot be—
and usually is not—sustained unless the diet is strictly
followed. Most people, especially those with few or no

symptoms, are not willing to make the severe alterations in life-style that such a diet demands.

Medication does not help everyone with a cholesterol and/or triglyceride problem. Some respond better than others, and, of course, all of the drugs may have some side effects.

Nicotinic acid, for instance, one of the oldest drugs used for this purpose, causes flushing of the skin in nearly all patients when they start taking it, and this persists in 10 to 15 percent. Some people experience gastrointestinal disturbances or show alteration in skin pigmentation. A more serious—but less frequent—reaction is impairment of liver function, including jaundice.

Cholestyramine can cause constipation, although there are no other known side effects of the drug. However, its effectiveness is limited. Reports on its results range from a 2 percent to a 43 percent reduction in cholesterol levels, and there are patients who do not respond at all.

Response often depends on the specific type of hyperlipidemia involved and on patient compliance.

Clofibrate, the drug used most often to reduce blood lipids, has few side effects but may cause nausea in 5 percent of those who take it, and there is a possibility of a relationship to the development of abnormal liver function.

A six-year study on 350 patients on clofibrate, compared to 367 patients taking a placebo (a substance with no expected therapeutic value), showed that clofibrate seemed to decrease patient mortality and prevent acute cardiac events (heart attack, increased intensity of angina if the patient had pre-existent angina). When the patients had had only a heart attack with no angina, clofibrate seemed to have no significant effect.

Dr. Buchwald believes that "clofibrate may show effective reductions in both serum [blood] cholesterol and serum triglyceride concentrations [in certain types of patients]. But those who respond well comprise only a small number of patients with high blood lipid levels." For the majority of people with hyperlipidemia, he feels that clofibrate is effective in lowering triglycerides, but significantly less so in reducing cholesterol.

There were 66 males and 35 females, ranging in age from 7 to 63 in the first 101 patients operated on for partial ileal bypass at the University of Minnesota. Eighty-one had evidence of coronary heart disease and were referred to Minnesota for surgery to manage their hyperlipidemia. All patients were put on special low-fat diets for at least three months before surgery.

Over a seven-year follow-up period, the average reduction in blood cholesterol levels was 40 percent from the level prior to surgery, but after three months of low-cholesterol dieting. The drop in cholesterol remained stable with the passage of time.

In this same study, fifteen patients with alarmingly elevated triglyceride levels experienced dramatic reductions, from 1,200 to 531 mg. percent.

Dr. Buchwald and other studies which report similar results note that some patients say they have experienced improvement in the symptoms of angina since surgery and are able to tolerate increased exercise without chest pain or other symptoms.

The Minnesota series describes ninety-four patients, thirty-nine of whom did not have angina before surgery and fifty-five who did. Of the thirty-nine patients without symptoms, none developed angina after the operation. Of the fifty-five who had angina prior to surgery, 7 percent said they felt worse, 24 percent experienced no change, 25 percent felt moderately improved, 18 percent felt dramatically better and 26 percent had total remission of angina. In conclusion, 69 percent of patients with angina before surgery had some degree of improvement afterward.

However, this testimony is not conclusive; it is hoped that the results of the current POSCH study will be the definitive ones.

"Most people who enter the POSCH study are not candidates for coronary bypass surgery at this time," says Dr. William L. Holmes, chairman of research at the Lankenau Medical Research Center. "Because their atherosclerosis is relatively stable, they are not severely symptomatic and they have done well on stress tests. When we explain that the disease is progressive, they feel that the partial ileal bypass is their best chance to keep it from accelerating."

"Many people enter the study because they have a desire to be at the forefront of medical therapy and hope also to improve their personal health status," says Lankenau's Dr. Sawin. "In addition, they and their doctors believe in the lipid-atherosclerosis hypothesis [the theory that it is high levels of blood fats that cause the development of atherosclerosis]."

Patients who participate in the study will be recruited at least until May 1983, but the eligibility requirements are strict. They must be between thirty and sixty-four years old and have had only one heart attack, experienced in the five years prior to enrollment in the study. Their total blood cholesterol levels must exceed 220 (or 200 if the LDL—low-density lipoproteins—are 140 or more on a diet designed to lower lipids), and they must not weigh more than 40 percent above their ideal weight as published in the Metropolitan Life Insurance Tables. Their systolic blood pressure must be less than 180, and their diastolic less than 105 without medication. Patients must not have had coronary artery or other heart surgery and must be free of any other disease, such as malignancy, chronic pulmonary insufficiency, thyroid disease, etc., that might make long-term survival unlikely. In addition, patients must be willing to be randomized either to standard medical or surgical treatment.

If at the conclusion of the study it becomes apparent that surgery does lead to reduction of atherosclerosis through lowering cholesterol, medical patients who want it will be offered the operation.

All patients—medical and surgical—will be followed for at least five years after randomization and will have full medical evaluations periodically.

During the project's course, the following incidents will be documented:

- sudden death;
- death due to atherosclerotic disease;
- acute heart attack;
- development of—or change in—existent angina;
- stroke;
- transient strokes;
- aortic aneurysm (a scarred area of the heart that holds blood);
- intermittent claudication (pain in the leg vessels after walking certain distances);
- congestive heart failure;
- progressive enlargement of the heart.

In addition, changes in exercise performance will be noted; later in the study, patients' coronary arteries will be re-evaluated through coronary arteriography.

"Recruitment of patients is tedious and difficult," says Helene Brooks, Lankenau's project coordinator, "because the criteria for entering the project are so exquisite. We want this study to be definitive and unimpeachable so we can prove, or disprove, once and for all, that lowering cholesterol retards or regresses the progression of atherosclerosis. We believe we will prove that it does."

Eleanor S. had always believed in health foods, dietary supplements and vitamins, and she was impressed with an article she once read which described a formula said to be helpful in combating heart disease. However, she paid little attention to it until several years later, when her husband, a photographer for a metropolitan newspaper, suffered a heart attack. Benjamin had never been ill before, nor had he exhibited any signs of heart disease. But while he was in the hospital, his wife's memory shot back to the article she had read several years earlier. It described the experience of Dr. Jacobus Rinse, a Dutch-American research chemist who was stricken with angina more than a quarter of a century ago and decided to seek a cure for his condition.

He developed a combination of natural-food elements that, he says, if consumed in the correct proportions, seems to remove the cholesterol deposits in the vessels. His ingredients include lecithin, linoleate oil, brewer's yeast, wheat germ, bone meal, vitamins and brown sugar in yogurt. After swallowing this mixture once a day for several months, Dr. Rinse says his angina vanished.

The formula, a dry granular mixture known as Dr. Rinse's Breakfast, is sold in some health-food stores in this country and has been written about in a variety of health publications often displayed in those stores. Doctors interviewed for this book either had never heard of the formula or did not know enough about it to comment.

Nonetheless, Eleanor prepares it every morning for herself and her husband. She mixes two tablespoons of lecithin granules, one tablespoon of brewer's yeast, one teaspoon of bone meal, one tablespoon of wheat germ and a tablespoon of oil. She mixes it with milk, cereal and a sliced banana. "It doesn't taste terrific," she admits, "but if it is helping, you learn to get used to it."

Eleanor acknowledges that she and her husband really do not know whether swallowing this mixture is helping at all. But so far, there has been no recurrence of heart problems, so they are planning to continue using it. "It doesn't seem to be hurting," she says, "so we might as well stick with it."

Most doctors interviewed, while they doubted it would do any substantial good, nevertheless agreed that it probably wouldn't do any harm, either.

≡ EPILOGUE

The death rate from heart attacks in the United States has dropped 25 percent in the past ten years. Most physicians feel confident that the decline will continue because of the coronary bypass operation, more efficient use of beta-blockers, the introduction of new drugs such as the calcium antagonists and the vigorous attempt to reduce the risk factors associated with atherosclerosis.

Expectation is growing that increased numbers of heart patients will be able to be controlled with drugs and alterations in their life-styles. A significant number, however, will continue to need bypass surgery to relieve their pain and, perhaps, to prolong their lives.

Informed patients should discuss their options with their physicians. Most doctors, recognizing that there can be dramatic variance in the way different practitioners will treat the same condition, encourage a "second opinion," and patients should not be timid about seeking one.

If a patient's physician has the reputation for being conservative, it might be wise to check with someone more aggressive. If a physician is known to be radical in his or her treatment of heart disease, a more moderate practitioner should be consulted. *Patients are entitled to know all of their options.*

No matter the course of treatment prescribed, patients have the right to ask tough, direct questions. More physicians should welcome patients who want information that will help them pursue their medical care intelligently.

In the end, many patients admit that what they decide to do is based on a "gut feeling" and confidence in a specific doctor, a faith that he or she will make them well. But more patients are recognizing that blind faith is not enough.

"In the final analysis, it is the judgment, wisdom, experience and skill of the doctors in whom a patient places his confidence, that count most heavily in determining the course of treatment," says Dr. Isadore Rosenfeld, clinical professor of medicine at the New York Hospital–Cornell Medical Center, and the author of *Second Opinion.* "But such confidence will be justified when the patient acts from a position of knowledge as well as faith."

APPENDIX I:
THE MAJOR STUDIES

No operation in the history of medicine has grown in popularity and accelerated in frequency of performance as rapidly as has heart-bypass surgery.

In the beginning, the operation was performed only on those persons whose angina could not be relieved by medical management. But as it became clear through the increased use of angiograms that a person's symptoms often had no relationship to the extent or danger of his disease, bypass surgery was recommended even for those with no symptoms or mild symptoms.

At first, reservations about the operation were confined to medical circles, and the undercurrent of skepticism about putting into widespread use a serious operation that had not yet proven itself was an "in-house" matter. Recently, however, the controversy has surfaced publicly, and there is greater awareness of significant differences of opinion among respected physicians and surgeons about the value of the operation.

Critics struggle with the answers to complex questions:

- Who will benefit most from bypass surgery?
- Is it true that large numbers of people could be managed as well or better through medical treatment?
- Will the operation prevent a heart attack?
- Will it induce one?
- Is the surgery riskier than the disease?

- Will it prolong life?
- Or is it a procedure that has gotten out of hand, promoted by opportunistic cardiac surgeons who are more concerned about the size of their bank accounts than the survival of their patients?

In a scathing editorial written for the *New England Journal of Medicine,* Dr. Eugene Braunwald of the Harvard Medical School and Peter Bent Brigham Hospital in Boston says, "An increasing number of patients are being operated upon, not because of the presence of intractable angina pectoris, a situation in which the efficacy of the procedure is not in dispute, but because of the hope, largely without objective supporting evidence at present, that coronary artery bypass surgery prolongs life or diminishes the frequency of subsequent myocardial infarction (or accomplishes both)."

A London physician, Dr. Attilio Maseri, who delivered the twenty-fifth annual James B. Herrick Memorial Lecture to the Chicago Heart Association in 1981, said that "many bypass patients could probably be treated just as well and at a fraction of the cost with new drugs."

Dr. W. Dudley Johnson of the Medical College of Wisconsin argues that people without any signs of heart disease are experiencing heart attacks and sudden death every day because of blocked arteries. If those arteries were bypassed, he reasons, their risk of death would diminish considerably.

The controversy is far from settled. But efforts to do so proliferate. Most major medical centers which perform bypass surgery have undertaken their own studies to compare patients treated medically and those treated surgically. And there have been a number of larger, cooperative studies (those in which several institutions participated) which have randomized patients to either surgical or medical treatment and then compared results.

As pointed out in Chapter 4, there have been criticisms of every kind of study, and there is no precisely perfect way to compare the effects of bypass surgery with medical treatment. And since the operation is relatively new, study results are limited and cannot predict long-range [beyond 10 years] outcome.

Moreover, the studies sometimes produce contradictory results, which add more confusion than enlightenment. And there is a feeling that studies orchestrated by surgical teams at leading medical centers are biased toward surgery.

Nonetheless, the information revealed in the studies offers clues, based on past—though limited—experience, about who benefits most from the bypass operation and why this is so.

The Major Studies

I. A RANDOMIZED STUDY CONDUCTED BY THE
VETERANS ADMINISTRATION ON THE TREATMENT OF
PATIENTS WITH CHRONIC STABLE ANGINA

This condition is angina over a long period of time—at least six months—which has not changed in intensity and is controlled through medical management. The results of the study were published in September 1977 in the *New England Journal of Medicine.*

The study was developed in 1970, as a cooperative effort, to determine the efficacy of the bypass operation in persons with *chronic stable angina.* It evaluated 596 men, 310 of whom were placed at random into a group that was to be treated medically and 286 into a group that would receive surgery. All of the patients came from thirteen participating Veterans Administration hospitals.

All had chronic stable angina for at least six months, had suffered a heart attack more than six months before entering the study and had an acceptable ventricular function. Patients with disease of the left main coronary artery were excluded. Those in both groups were remarkably similar in characteristics and risk factors except for cholesterol levels (more medical patients had cholesterol levels lower than 249).

The findings were:

· Operative mortality (within 30 days of surgery) averaged 5.6 percent. There were no deaths in patients with one-vessel disease; six deaths among those with two-vessel disease and nine deaths among patients with triple-vessel disease.

· Repeat angiograms, taken from ten months to thirty-six months after surgery, showed that an average of 69 percent of the grafts were still open. Fifty-four percent of patients had all of their bypass grafts open; 12 percent had all grafts closed; and 88 percent had at least one graft open.

· Seventy-seven patients (from both medical and surgical groups) died during the observation period, which ranged from twenty-one to thirty-six months. In the medical group, 82 percent of the deaths occurred because of cardiac problems; 88 percent of the surgical patients died of cardiac causes, but 56 percent of those were considered surgical deaths (they occurred at or within thirty days of surgery).

· *At thirty-six months, survival of the medical group was 87 percent; and survival in the surgical group was 88 percent, an insignificant difference.* Patients with double-vessel disease and an abnormal left ventricle had a survival rate of 84 percent after three years, whether they were treated medically or surgically.

Patients who had abnormal left ventricles and triple-vessel disease showed an 82 percent survival if treated medically and 86 percent if treated surgically.

The report, which was considered significant because it was the first major randomized study in which several medical centers cooperated, concluded that *"there was no statistical difference in survival between medically and surgically treated cohorts . . ."*

However, large numbers of cardiologists and cardiac surgeons attacked it as unreliable and misleading. They protested that:

· Surgical mortality was higher than in almost any other study.
· The average number of bypass grafts per patient was well under the number of diseased arteries, thus leaving the patient with arteries still clogged.
· Six percent of patients per year dropped out of the medical group and had surgery.
· Only low-risk patients were included.
· The criterion of 50 percent blockages is less than in most other studies which require that blockages be at least 70 percent.
· The quality of coronary angiograms was poor; therefore, determination of the size and degree of blockages was chancy.

Nonetheless, Dr. Thomas C. Chalmers and his colleagues at the Mount Sinai School of Medicine in New York defend the study and suggest that mortality rates in the VA study are excessive only if compared to the very low mortality statistics in a few isolated centers. Further, they stated that the study is a "well-done randomized control study."

And Boston's Dr. Eugene Braunwald says that "even if

the operative mortality had been lower (in the VA study) and the survivors of the operation had followed the same survival curve as the patients described in the study, *it would be difficult for the surgical results to be substantially better than those of medical treatment, so far as longevity is concerned, simply because the medically treated group exhibited a cumulative survival of eighty-seven percent at thirty-six months, a mortality rate approximating only four percent per year."*

Dr. Braunwald points out that all the patients had symptoms and that the incidences of left ventricular abnormality and multivessel disease were high. He also comments that just as the results of surgical treatment have improved, "medical therapy has not stood still either."

Only about two-thirds of the patients randomized to medical therapy in the VA study received propranolol, because this beta-blocker was not approved for treatment of angina until midway through the patient-selection portion of the VA study. (The patients were not treated, of course, with the newer calcium antagonists, which are still not approved for general use in this country.) Dr. Braunwald believes that if beta-blockers improve the survival of patients with coronary artery disease, "it will be less likely that surgical treatment will materially improve the survival of most patients with coronary artery disease."

Dr. M. L. Murphy, chief of cardiology at Little Rock Veterans Administration Hospital and the University of Arkansas Medical Center, is senior author of the Veterans Administration study. He agrees that some of the criticism may be valid but says, "This report was intended to be preliminary, and it reflects what was happening at that time. Following the criticism, we reanalyzed our data to include the ten Veterans Administration centers with mortality rates comparable to other leading centers at the time—three point six percent—and we still came up with the same results. We recognize that surgical procedures have advanced, but so have medical procedures, and there is a need for continued studies."

II. THE VA COOPERATIVE RANDOMIZED STUDY OF SURGERY FOR CORONARY ARTERIAL OCCLUSIVE DISEASE: SUBGROUP WITH SIGNIFICANT LEFT MAIN LESION.

Results of the study were published in *Circulation* in December 1976. Senior author was Dr. Timothy Takaro of the Veterans Administration Hospital in Asheville, North Carolina.

A subgroup of 113 patients with disease of the left main coronary artery was culled from the larger Veterans Administration study and analyzed in the first randomized prospective controlled trial (see Chapter 4) on patients with this characteristic.

The average age of the patients in the medical group was fifty-four and in the surgical group was fifty-two. Risk factors were approximately equal between the groups.

Results showed that:

· Two patients randomized to medical care died within one month.
· Operative mortality (death within thirty days of surgery) was 14 percent, but that figure was higher in the first two years of the study and dropped dramatically in the final three years.
· *The survival rate of surgically randomized patients was significantly better than medically randomized patients at eighteen, twenty-four and thirty months.* At thirty-six months, however, the difference be-

tween the two groups decreased because two surgical patients died during that time.

- High-risk patients—those with triple-vessel disease, with one vessel being the left main artery, and abnormal left ventricular function—did significantly better with surgery than with medical treatment.

III. PROSPECTIVE RANDOMIZED STUDY OF CORONARY ARTERY BYPASS SURGERY IN STABLE ANGINA PECTORIS: SURVIVAL AT TWO YEARS.

This is known as the European Cooperative Study and was published in the *Lancet,* September 6, 1980.

Investigators from 12 European countries participated in a prospective controlled study (see Chapter 4), which included 768 men under 65 with angina, at least 50 percent obstruction in two or more coronary arteries and ejection fractions of more than 50 percent (normal).

The patients were admitted into the study between September 1973 and March 1976, and were randomized to either surgery or medical care. Patients in both groups were similar in risk factors and in duration of angina.

Medical treatment varied from center to center and was not standardized. It was based on the judgment of the physician and continued for as long as it was indicated.

Results of a three-year follow-up for all patients and three- to five-year follow-up for some showed that:

- Surgery was associated with a significantly better five-year survival than that of no surgery, the rates being 93.5 percent for the surgical patients and 84.1 percent for the medical group.
- Patients with left main disease had a 92.9 percent five-year survival when treated surgically and a 61.7 percent five-year survival when treated medically.

- Patients with three-vessel disease also benefitted from surgery. More than 94 percent of those who had operations were alive after five years compared with almost 85 percent in the group that did not.
- Symptoms and exercise tolerance were improved for those in the surgical group.
- Fifty-two patients in the medical group and 25 in the surgical group have died.
- Operative mortality was 3.5 percent for 456 operations.
- No significant difference between the two survival curves was found in the subgroup of patients with two-vessel disease (the study showed that the remarkably good survival in medical patients with two-vessel disease may be associated with a left anterior descending coronary artery (LAD) that is *not* blocked. In 40 percent of medical patients in this group, the LAD was not obstructed, and survival was 96 percent at 60 months. In the remaining 60 percent where the LAD was blocked, survival was 82 percent.
- The greatest difference between the two groups was the proportion of symptom-free patients. At one, two and three years, the proportions of patients without symptoms were 58, 55 and 49 percent for the surgical group and 15, 16 and 20 percent for the medical group.

It is difficult to compare results of the VA and European studies because the VA study included patients who were older, had single-vessel disease and who had lower ejection fractions. Operative mortality was different also: in the European study, it was 3.5 percent compared with 5.6 percent for the VA study for patients with single-, double- or triple-vessel disease.

IV. UNSTABLE ANGINA PECTORIS: NATIONAL
COOPERATIVE STUDY GROUP TO COMPARE SURGICAL
AND MEDICAL THERAPY. IN-HOSPITAL EXPERIENCE
AND INITIAL FOLLOW-UP RESULTS IN PATIENTS WITH
ONE-, TWO- AND THREE-VESSEL DISEASE.

The results of this prospective randomized study, in
which nine medical centers cooperated under the auspices of the National Heart, Lung, and Blood Institute,
were published in the November 1978 issue of the *American Journal of Cardiology.* All patients were suffering
from unstable angina, a virulent form of angina said to
precede myocardial infarction (heart attack), or even sudden death. Although there have been a few studies comparing medical and surgical therapy for this condition,
none has resolved the controversy.

Patients who entered the study were all under seventy
and had unstable angina severe enough to require hospitalization to determine whether they were indeed experiencing heart attacks. All had blockages of at least 70
percent in one, two or three coronary arteries.

Those assigned to medical therapy received propranolol and long-acting nitrates in the doses needed to
achieve control of blood pressure and pulse throughout a
twenty-four-hour period. A systolic blood pressure of 110
to 120 and a pulse rate of about 60 were considered adequate.

Results showed that:

· *The overall in-hospital mortality rate* was 3 percent
for medical patients and 5 percent for surgical patients. Patients with disease of one coronary artery had
an in-hospital mortality rate of 6 percent if they were
treated medically and no mortalities if they were
treated surgically; patients with three-vessel disease

had no in-hospital mortalities if they were in the medical group and 10 percent if they were randomized to surgery.

- At one-year follow-up, the *survival rate* for medical patients was 93 percent, and for surgical patients it was 92 percent. At two years, survival rates were 91 percent for medical patients and 90 percent for surgical patients. But 36 percent of medically treated patients later had surgery because their angina had become too severe.

- The rate of nonfatal *heart attack in the hospital* was similar for medical and surgical patients with one-vessel disease but was higher for patients who had two- and three-vessel disease when they underwent surgery. The overall in-hospital rate of heart attack was 17 percent for all patients treated with surgery, compared with 8 percent for all patients treated medically.

- The rate of *nonfatal heart attack after release from the hospital* was higher in surgical patients than in medically treated patients when they had either one or two blockages. But it was higher in medically treated patients when they had obstruction of three arteries. The overall rate of nonfatal heart attacks during the follow-up period was 11 percent in medical patients and 13 percent in surgical patients.

- *Severe angina* during the follow-up period was much more common in patients under medical care than in those who had received surgery.

- Of the fifty-three *patients randomized to medical care who later had surgery,* 20 percent had one-vessel disease; 33 percent had two-vessel disease; and 49 percent had three-vessel disease. The number of vessels involved seemed to be the only feature that correlated with the patient's subsequent need for surgery.

- *Second operation for angina* incompatible with the patient's life-style was performed on five patients—two with disease of one artery, two with disease of two arteries and one with three-vessel disease.
- Approximately 70 percent of patients with disease of one or two coronary arteries *returned to work* during the first two years, no matter whether they were treated medically or surgically. So did 50 percent of those with three-vessel disease, regardless of the treatment received.
- Because of improved surgical techniques and management, the rates of in-hospital mortality and heart attack varied dramatically from the early to the late years of the study.

The investigators concluded that:

- Coronary bypass surgery can be performed in patients with unstable angina, with reasonable safety and good clinical results.
- Intensive medical therapy is an acceptable alternative to urgent bypass surgery because the rates of in-hospital mortality and heart attack are lower than they were once thought to be.
- After a thirty-month follow-up period, it was found that medical therapy had been effective in the majority of patients. But more medically than surgically treated patients suffered from severe angina.
- Patients with more extensive coronary artery blockages are more likely to need surgery later because their angina has interfered with their life-style.
- Rate of survival for persons treated medically was higher in this cooperative study than it had been in studies reported earlier; the investigators believe that a reasonable explanation may be the improvement in medical therapy in recent years, namely the use of beta-blockers and long-acting nitrates.

V. UNSTABLE ANGINA PECTORIS: NATIONAL
COOPERATIVE STUDY GROUP TO COMPARE SURGICAL
AND MEDICAL THERAPY: [RESULTS IN PATIENTS WITH
ST SEGMENT ELEVATION DURING PAIN].

This study included 79 of the original 288 patients in the
cooperative study under the auspices of the National
Heart, Lung, and Blood Institute, whose pain at rest was
associated with changes on electrocardiograms, namely
elevations—transient, not permanent—of the critical ST
segment. Elevations, rather than depressions, of ST segment have been called "variant" or Prinzmetal's angina
and indicate that angina may be caused by spasm, rather
than—or in addition to—blocked coronary arteries. Forty-
two patients were treated medically and 37 had urgent
bypass surgery. Results were reported in the April 1980
issue of the *American Journal of Cardiology.*

The *overall mortality rate* (including those who died in
the hospital) *was 7 percent for the medical and 16 percent
for the surgical group at the end of forty-two months.*
This was not significantly different from the survival rate
of patients who did not demonstrate elevation of ST segment during pain episodes.

Of those who survived the forty-two-month follow-up
period, 6 percent of those treated medically and 10 percent of those treated surgically had heart attacks, comparable to the 7 percent rate of heart attack for medically
treated and 15 percent for surgically treated patients who
did not have ST segment elevations.

There was a dramatic difference, however, in the incidence of severe angina between the group with ST elevations and the group free of them. For instance, in the
first and second years of the follow-up period, 10 percent of medical patients and 15 percent of surgical patients with ST segment elevations complained of severe
angina. But 41 percent of the medically treated and 10

percent of the surgically treated patients without the ST
segment elevation suffered intense angina during the
same period.

*The investigators conclude that "patients with unstable
angina pectoris associated with ST segment elevation during episodes of pain can be stabilized and managed with
a maximal medical program consisting of nitrites, long-
acting nitrates and propranolol in dosages that achieve
therapeutic control of blood pressure and pulse rate. Medical therapy is successful in most cases. . . . Later, if intensive medical therapy has failed, the patient can undergo
more elective surgery with no increase in risk over that of
patients who received early urgent surgery."*

VI. SURGICAL TREATMENT OF CORONARY ARTERY DISEASE

This is a prospective study of the first 1,000 patients operated on between September 1969 and June 1974 at the
Montreal Heart Institute to determine the fate of the
grafts that were inserted and the effect on symptoms and
on survival. Senior author was Dr. Lucien Campeau, and
the results were published in *Medicine North America,*
September 1980.

They showed that:

- A few grafts became closed after the first year of surgery, the annual attrition rate being 0.7 percent in
  patients operated on in the later years of the study.
  During the first year after surgery whether or not the
  graft remained open had a lot to do with the quality
  of the "distal runoff" (the portion of the artery beyond
  the blockage).
- New blockages of 50 percent or more, or blockages in
  the segment of the artery beyond the graft, were

found in only 3.2 percent of the grafted arteries studied. Thus, the investigators concluded that bypass surgery does not promote atherosclerosis in the distal coronary artery, as had been feared when this surgery was initiated.

- After twelve years of experience, relief of angina is the *only* objective of bypass surgery that has been fully realized. The study showed that, during the first few years, 70–90 percent of patients experienced relief of symptoms and that the operation was more effective than medical treatment. During the subsequent three to six years, angina recurs at the rate of approximately 10 percent a year, the main causes being changes in arteries that had not been bypassed, changes in grafted arteries and the natural progression of atherosclerosis.
- Except for the relief of pain, the only noncontroversial indication for bypass surgery is the necessity to graft a blockage in the left main coronary artery in the hope of prolonging survival.
- Surgery is indicated in asymptomatic young patients when they have severe triple-vessel coronary disease, especially if there is a family history of heart disease and premature death, and evidence of atherosclerosis as shown by a stress test or thallium scan.
- Patients with triple-vessel disease and stable angina may have increased life span if they undergo surgery.

The report from the Montreal Heart Institute emphasizes that "controversy still reigns over the entire chapter of preventive surgery or surgery based solely on the hope of increasing survival. When such surgery is contemplated, the following angiographic criteria become mandatory; severe narrowing of at least 70 percent, excellent distal runoff [good arteries beyond the blockages], good left ventricular contraction and the possibility of complete correction."

VII. SURVIVAL PATTERNS IN LEFT MAIN CORONARY DISEASE SUBSETS: RESULTS OF THE CASS STUDY.

The aim of this study, in which fifteen institutions participated (see Chapter 4), was to evaluate survival in patients with left main coronary artery disease when they were treated medically and surgically. The results were reported by Dr. Bernard R. Chaitman at the Fifty-third Annual Scientific Sessions of the American Heart Association in Miami Beach, November 1980.

Of 1,492 patients with a greater than 50 percent blockage of their left main coronary artery, 1,183 had bypass surgery. The others were treated medically. Both groups, however, were similar with respect to age, gender, history of heart attack, extent of disease and risk factors. But the group that received surgery had more severe angina, required more medication and had more serious blockages of the left main coronary artery. Their left ventricular function, however, was a little better than that of their medical counterparts.

At the end of four years, 88 percent of the surgical group, but only 63 percent of the medical group, was alive. Older patients did not do as well as younger ones. The older patient (over sixty-five) had only a 51 percent chance of being alive in four years when treated medically, but 82 percent of the surgical group in that age range survived at least forty-eight months.

The survival rate had a lot to do with the patient's left ventricular function, but no matter the degree of left ventricular function, the surgical group did better.

The CASS research concluded that "coronary bypass

surgery prolongs life in most patients with left main coronary disease, especially those with severe left main coronary narrowing or impaired left ventricular function.

"In nonoperated patients with left main coronary disease, the most important determinants of survival are the percent of left main stenosis [blockage], left ventricular score [a measurement of left ventricular function based on several factors], age and existence of hypertension.

"In patients with left main coronary disease who undergo coronary bypass surgery, the most important determinants of long-term survival are preoperative left ventricular function, age and coronary dominance.

VIII. COMPARISONS OF THE EFFECTS ON SURVIVAL AFTER CORONARY ARTERY SURGERY IN SUBGROUPS OF PATIENTS FROM THE SEATTLE HEART WATCH.

The Seattle Heart Watch is a community-wide registry of 2,616 patients from all laboratories that performed coronary angiography between 1969 and 1974. Of the 1,533 patients in this study, 1,158 were treated surgically, and 375 were treated medically. The study's purpose was to compare the effects on survival between the two groups.

This is what the study revealed:

· Patients who seemed most likely to benefit by enhanced survival from surgery were those over the age of forty-eight, with two- or three-vessel disease, normal or moderately normal ejection fraction (more than 30 percent) and no history of congestive heart failure.

· Younger patients (under forty-eight) do not benefit as much from surgery as older patients. In fact, patients younger than forty-eight with one-vessel disease or a history of congestive heart failure did better when treated medically.

· The effect of surgery was *not significant* in any age group for persons with one-vessel disease and even carried a higher risk for patients under forty-eight who received surgery.

· Persons with less severe angina benefitted more from surgery although patients with all degrees of angina were helped significantly.

· Patients with three-vessel disease had enhanced survival when they received surgery.

X. EFFECT OF CORONARY SURGERY ON SURVIVAL IN ASYMPTOMATIC AND MINIMALLY SYMPTOMATIC PATIENTS.

This study, part of the Seattle Heart Watch (described above) measured the effect on survival of 277 medically treated and 392 surgically treated patients who had surgery for coronary artery disease that was producing no or few symptoms, but who had at least one major artery with a 70 or greater percent blockage. Senior author is Dr. K.E. Hammermeister, and results were reported in *Circulation* in August 1980.

Results showed that:

· Fifteen of 392 patients died at surgery or before discharge from the hospital (two with one-vessel disease and eight with two-vessel disease).

· Significantly improved survival was seen only in the group with three-vessel disease.

· Those with two-vessel disease showed slight but statistically insignificant improvement in survival with surgery.

- Patients with one-vessel disease survived as well with medical therapy as they did with surgery.
- Ejection fraction was the most important predictor of survival.

The investigators do not, despite their findings, recommend prophylactic bypass surgery for all patients who have three-vessel disease. They feel that persons with significant distal-vessel disease (blockages all the way to the end of the artery), severe left ventricular dysfunction or other major medical disease would probably not benefit. Even more important, they say that "patients with ejection fractions of more than fifty-one percent have excellent prognosis regardless of treatment; therefore, for this group, it would seem prudent to wait until significant symptoms develop before recommending surgery."

XI. PROGRESS STUDY OF 590 CONSECUTIVE NONSURGICAL CASES OF CORONARY DISEASE FOLLOWED 5–9 YEARS.

This study (senior author is Dr. Albert V. G. Bruschke) traces the natural history of patients with coronary artery disease who were treated medically during the years that bypass was not routinely used. It is considered critical because it is the study which is traditionally compared with results of surgery. It is important to note, however, that since this report was issued, medical treatment of patients has improved dramatically . . . so comparing current surgical results against medical treatment of a decade ago may not yield valid information.

The progress of 590 patients whose coronary arteriograms showed significant blockages was followed for five to nine years.

Results showed that:

The two factors which correlated most closely with incidence of mortality were the function of the left ventricle and the number of vessels involved.

As could be expected, mortality was lowest (seven deaths out of one hundred patients) where only one vessel was diseased and the left ventricle was normal. It was highest where there was blockage in three vessels or in the left main coronary artery and there was a poorly functioning left ventricle.

At the end of five years, 23 percent of patients with one-vessel disease, 38 percent of those with two-vessel disease, 54 percent of those with triple-vessel disease and 57 percent of those with obstruction of the left main coronary artery had died.

The mortality, when the function of the left ventricle was considered, was 25 percent at the end of five years for those with a normal ventricle, and 69 percent for those with the worst-functioning left ventricles.

Patients who had congestive heart failure were at increased risk of death.

Findings on the electrocardiogram also figured heavily in predicting mortality. Only 18.7 percent of patients with normal electrocardiograms died during the follow-up period, but there was a 65.1 percent death rate among those with conduction disturbances on the electrocardiogram.

XII. THE AORTOCORONARY BYPASS OPERATION: MYTH AND REALITY. AN OVERVIEW BASED ON 10,000 OPERATIONS AT THE TEXAS HEART INSTITUTE.

This study, which was published in *International Surgery* in 1978, looked at more than 10,000 patients who received coronary artery bypass surgery at the Texas Heart

Institute between 1968 and the end of 1977. Senior author is Frank M. Sandiford.

These were the results:

· Death in the hospital (either during surgery or before discharge) declined as the study continued. During 1970, hospital mortality was 9.1 percent; in 1977, it was 1.5 percent.
· There were more hospital deaths among women than men. During 1977, the last year of the study, hospital mortality of men was reduced to 1.1 percent, but in females to only 4.2 percent.
· A long-term follow-up (from 24 to 96 months) showed that 92 percent of those who survived were free of pain or significantly improved.
· The cumulative survival of the group was 91.7 percent at the end of three years, 87.7 percent at the end of five years and 79.6 percent at the end of eight years.

XIII. DOES CORONARY SURGERY PROLONG LIFE IN COMPARISON WITH MEDICAL MANAGEMENT?

This study (senior author is Dr. Robert A. Rosati), conducted by the Division of Cardiology, Department of Medicine and Department of Community Health Sciences at Duke University Medical Center, was published in *Postgraduate Medical Journal* in 1976. The analysis considers Duke University Medical Center's series of *concurrent* operated and nonoperated patients to determine whether bypass surgery prolongs life in comparison to medical management.

The analysis was made on 1,101 consecutive patients with coronary artery disease who were catheterized at Duke between August 1969 and September 1974. All had blockages of 70 percent or more. The patients were followed up at six months, one year and annually thereafter up to five years. Of the group, 490 patients had surgery, and 611 were treated medically. Of those 611, 21 were operated on more than six months after their first catheterization.

At the end of four years, the survival rate for surgically treated patients was 82 percent and for medical patients was 78 percent, rates considered not to be substantially different.

The investigators conclude that "it is probable that for the average patient with coronary artery disease, bypass surgery does not significantly prolong life over a 4-year period."

However, they believe that follow-up over long periods of time will be necessary before it can be determined whether or not survival is affected by surgery.

XIV. OUTCOME IN MEDICALLY TREATED CORONARY ARTERY DISEASE: ISCHEMIC EVENTS: NONFATAL INFARCTION AND DEATH.

This study, which considered the outcome of 1,214 medically treated patients with coronary artery disease at Duke University Medical Center, was published in *Circulation* in 1980. Senior author is Dr. Phillip J. Harris.

All of the patients had angina, and all were treated with short-acting nitrates, dietary advice and treatment to reduce their risk factors. As soon as they were available, long-acting nitrates and beta-blocking agents were also used.

These were the results:

- There were, at the end of seven years, 245 deaths from cardiac causes and 14 deaths from other causes.
- There were 128 nonfatal heart attacks, but 28 of those patients who had them died later.

Significant predictors of nonfatal heart attack or death were

- the degree of heart failure;
- the number of diseased arteries;
- progressive chest pain;
- the presence of Prinzmetal's angina (angina caused by spasm);
- extremely abnormal left ventricular contraction;
- significant disease of the left main coronary artery;
- history of peripheral vascular disease;
- abnormalities on a resting electrocardiogram;
- anterior left ventricular contraction abnormality;
- a poor cardiac output;
- chest pain at night.
- Although patients with multivessel disease and good left ventricular function have a high survival rate, they experience nonfatal heart attacks at the same rate as death. Since having a heart attack alters a person's prognosis, it is felt that improving the long-term survival rate in such patients may depend on reducing their incidence of heart attacks.

In conclusion, the authors consider that the natural history of persons with coronary artery disease is a series of "ischemic events" (cardiac events such as angina or heart attack, resulting from poor blood supply to the heart). Whether or not one survives an ischemic event is strongly influenced by the quality of the left ventricular function and the presence of disease of the left main coronary artery.

XV. BYPASS GRAFT SURGERY FOR CORONARY ARTERY DISEASE: A 10–13-YEAR STUDY OF 741 PATIENTS:

This study, which considered 741 consecutive patients who had bypass surgery at the Cleveland Clinic between

May 1967 and December 1970 and were followed for ten to thirteen years, was abstracted in the February 1981 issue of the *American Journal of Cardiology*.

There were 632 men and 109 women with a median age of 50. Sixty-nine patients had triple-vessel disease; 63 had left main disease; 414 had single-vessel disease; and 195 had double-vessel disease.

Results showed that:

- Twenty-two patients died in the hospital.
- Ninety-seven needed repeat bypass operations from 1 to 136 months after the original operation.
- One hundred thirty-two patients died from 2 to 135 months after being discharged from the hospital, but of these, at least 37 deaths were not from cardiac causes.
- Five-year survival rate for everyone entered in the study was 89.4 percent. Ten-year survival rate was 77.3 percent.
- For those with single-vessel disease, the five-year survival rate was 91.5 percent, and 81.3 percent at the end of ten years.
- Those with double-vessel disease showed a survival rate of 87.8 percent at the end of five years and 75.9 percent at the end of ten.
- Patients with triple-vessel blockages had a survival rate of 84.8 percent at five years and 62.3 percent at ten years.
- Left main disease patients had a survival rate of 85.5 percent after five years and 72.9 percent after ten years.

The doctors strongly believe that the use of four or more bypasses to reconstruct blood flow to all of the threatened coronary arteries is beneficial. They believe it is more effective not only in relieving angina, but in improving life expectancy.

XVI. THE NATURAL HISTORY OF ASYMPTOMATIC OR
MILDLY SYMPTOMATIC PATIENTS WITH CORONARY
ARTERY DISEASE.

Because coronary artery bypass surgery is increasingly being suggested to patients without symptoms (but have had poor stress test results, followed by angiograms which identified blocked arteries), or with mild symptoms, as a means of prolonging their lives, the Cardiology Branch of the National Heart, Lung, and Blood Institute of the National Institutes of Health conducted a study of these patients to determine whether surgery was justified. Chief investigator was Dr. Kenneth M. Kent, head of the Institute's Section on Cardiovascular Diagnosis.

The study considers the fact that bypass surgery seems justified (based on several studies) in such patients when results of the operation are compared to the natural-history studies (what happens without surgery) of similar patients during the 1960s and early 1970s. The purpose of this research was to determine whether the survival statistics of *today's* patients with mild or no symptoms would be different than those patients studied earlier; and how today's patients, with medical treatment now available, would compare in terms of survival to patients who do have surgery for coronary artery disease.

Included in the study were 147 men and women, ranging in age from 25 to 65. Persons with disease of the left main coronary artery or ejection fractions below 20 were eliminated.

All of the patients were followed (prospectively) from six to sixty-seven months. Results showed that:

- There were eight deaths in the total group during the follow-up period (a mortality rate of 3 percent a year).
- Mortality rate for triple-vessel disease was 6 percent a year; for single- and double-vessel disease it was 1.5 percent a year.
- Patients with triple-vessel disease who, despite mild symptoms, do poorly on exercise tests are at high risk. Of these, 20 percent died during the follow-up period, and another 20 percent developed symptoms severe enough to require surgery.
- Patients with triple-vessel disease who had good exercise capacity were at lower risk, with only 7 percent dying and 15 percent needing bypass surgery later. The annual mortality rate of these patients was 4 percent.
- Patients with one- or two-vessel disease, who have no symptoms or mild symptoms, have an excellent prognosis.

The investigators concluded that "because patients with three-vessel disease and poor exercise capacity have an extremely grave prognosis, it would appear reasonable to recommend coronary bypass operation, for this subgroup, even in the absence of supporting data derived from a definitive randomized study."

XVII. RESULTS OF CORONARY BYPASS AT LEAST 10 YEARS AFTER OPERATION IN 250 PATIENTS.

The goal of this study, undertaken at the Baylor College of Medicine in Houston, Texas, was to determine the outcome of the bypass operation in 250 patients who had operations between 1968 and 1971 and were followed for ten years. It is a significant study because of the long-term follow-up. Senior author is Dr. Gerald M. Lawrie.

The mean age of patients studied was 51.2 years. The largest number of patients (111) had disease of two coronary arteries; 58 patients had one-vessel disease, and 66 patients had blockages in three coronary arteries. Only 15 patients had a greater than 50 percent blockage in the left main coronary artery.

Ventricular function varied: 165 patients demonstrated good ventricular function . . . the rest were poor.

These were the results on 241 patients followed for a decade.

- Seventeen patients (6.8 percent) died at surgery or while in the hospital.
- Of patients with one-vessel disease, 40 patients (80 percent) with good left ventricular function were alive at ten years; 70 percent (5 patients) of those with poor left ventricular function were alive.
- Of patients with two-vessel disease, 48 patients (48 percent) with good left ventricular function were living at ten years; 28 patients (58 percent) with poor left ventricular function survived.
- Patients with three-vessel disease had a poorer outcome. Twenty-three of those with good left ventricular function (56 percent) were alive at ten years, and 12 patients (50 percent) with poor left ventricular function were alive.
- Nine patients with left main disease (60 percent) were living at the ten-year follow-up.

Between five and ten years after surgery, 77.4 percent of the grafts were open; and of 165 survivors, 58 percent had no symptoms. Twenty-six percent had improved symptoms, and 16 percent experienced no change in angina or complained of feeling worse.

Conclusions are: that the characteristics which best predicted survival were the patient's age, left ventricular function and the number of coronary arteries that were diseased before the operation.

XVIII. PROGNOSIS OF MEDICALLY TREATED PATIENTS WITH CORONARY-ARTERY DISEASE WITH PROFOUND ST-SEGMENT DEPRESSION DURING EXERCISE TESTING.

A person who demonstrates more than two millimeters depression in the vital ST-segment of an electrocardiograph during exercise testing is usually considered to be at significant risk because this finding has been associated with severe, multivessel coronary artery disease even if the patient has no symptoms. Patients who have this degree of ST depression when stress-tested are often sent for coronary angiograms and possible bypass surgery (even if they are symptom free).

This study, which was published November 5, 1981 in the *New England Journal of Medicine* (senior author is Dr. Philip J. Podrid), followed for 20 to 140 months 142 men with ST-segment depression provoked by exercise testing who did not have surgery, but whose symptoms were managed on a medical regimen. The men were from thirty-nine to eighty years old; all had had a prior heart attack or had angina or had had angiograms which showed coronary artery disease (two or three vessels were affected). All of the patients were treated with beta-blockers, long-acting nitrates and nitroglycerin, used prophylactically. All were placed on a diet and exercise program.

The 142 patients were divided into three groups, according to the stage they reached during exercise testing. Group one included 46 men who were able to exercise for an average of one to six minutes with ST changes occurring after 2.8 minutes. A follow-up of 52 months showed that:

- Four patients required bypass grafting because their angina could not be controlled with medical therapy.
- Of the 42 men continuing on medical therapy, four have died, an annual mortality rate of two percent.

Group two included patients who had exercised for six to nine minutes, with the ST change occurring after 4.6 minutes of exercise. After an average follow-up of 61 months, results showed that:

- Three patients have required bypass surgery.
- Of the 52 patients who continued with medical therapy, six have died, but one did not die of cardiac causes. Therefore, the annual cardiac mortality rate was 1.8 percent.

Group three consisted of 41 patients who exercised for longer than nine minutes, with the ST-segment depression coming on after five minutes of exercise. During the average follow-up period of 65 months, these were the results:

- Two patients required bypass surgery.
- Of the remaining 39 patients who were treated on medical therapy, there was only one death which was not from cardiac causes.

For the total group of 142 patients, there were heart attacks in three patients, and congestive heart failure developed in one patient after 36 months of follow-up.

In conclusion, the authors state: "It is common practice to refer patients with exercise-induced ST-segment depression of 2 mm or more to coronary angiography. The prevailing view is that such patients have far-advanced, multivessel involvement and high incidence of left main coronary artery disease or its equivalent. If such findings are confirmed, coronary-artery bypass operation is considered to be the only way to improve what otherwise is assumed to pose a dire outlook for survival.

"The importance of our study is that it provides evidence contesting this chain of reasoning. In fact, the finding of profound ST-segment depresssion after exercise testing is not associated with a poor prognosis. There is rarely a need to resort to cardiac surgery; medical management is highly successful and associated with a low mortality."

In evaluating the preceding studies, some of which produce conflicting findings, patients should be aware that it is often impossible to compare results from center to center, partly because surgical results are matched against non-current medical results.

It should also be remembered that comparing mortality figures from center to center is not as revealing as it may seem. Some centers will operate on patients with a higher degree of risk where the expected mortality is higher; others perform surgery primarily on low-risk patients. Therefore, a 1 or 2 percent hospital mortality rate may not be as impressive as it seems, depending on the condition of the surgical patients at that hospital or medical center.

In an effort to consider the status of coronary artery bypass surgery in 1980, the National Institutes of Health, the National Heart, Lung, and Blood Institute in conjunction with the National Center for Health Care Technology sponsored a conference to develop a consensus statement. The report issued is called the "National Institutes of Health Consensus Development Conference Statement on Coronary Artery Bypass Surgery: Scientific and Clinical Aspects." Conference chairman was Dr. Robert L. Frye, chairman of the division of cardiovascular diseases at the Mayo Clinic.

Conclusions reached were:

- Patients with severe blockages of the left main coronary artery or severe obstructions of multiple major coronary branches should seriously consider surgery.
- When medical therapy is initiated for a patient, it is critical to realize that an intensive effort is required by the physician, an effort which involves consideration of almost every aspect of the patient's life.
- Survivors of an acute heart attack are at high risk of sudden death during the first year after the attack; but several reports indicate that patients can be divided into high-risk and low-risk groups on the basis of their history, symptoms and noninvasive testing. High-risk patients should have coronary arteriography and angiography, to be followed by surgical intervention if the results indicate that it would be appropriate. However, there is not sufficient data to determine whether a bypass operation will reduce mortality.
- Comparison between medical and surgical therapy must consider the function of the patient's left ventricle, since this is critical to survival, as is the location and extent of the blockages.
- It seems unlikely that the benefits of surgery can be assessed from studies that are not adequately controlled (that are not compared with similar patients receiving medical therapy during the same period).
- Patients with angina who have more than a 50 percent blockage of the left main coronary artery will probably have a better chance of survival with surgery than with medical treatment. This is true regardless of left ventricular function or the degree of angina.
- Conflicting data exist on the most beneficial treatment for patients with three-vessel disease. Some studies

suggest that surgery improves survival in those patients with this condition, but who have good left ventricular ejection fraction (greater than 50 percent).
But it was felt that more investigaton is needed before
a definitive conclusion can be reached.

· The two large randomized studies (the VA and the
European Cooperative) do not find improved survival
with surgery in patients with two-vessel disease, no
matter the condition of the left ventricle.

· There is no evidence of improved survival after surgery in patients who have blockage in one coronary
artery, regardless of the status of the left ventricle.

· There is not enough information to support the premise that surgery enhances survival in patients with a
left ventricular ejection fraction of less than 20 percent.

· The randomized unstable angina trial, under the auspices of the National Heart, Lung, and Blood Institute,
did not show improved survival of patients treated by
urgent surgery compared to those treated by medical
management, unless the patient's symptoms were so
severe as to require an operation.

· Surgery may be appropriate for patients where large
areas of the heart are in jeopardy, even if there is not
unimpeachable evidence of improved survival.

· Angina is reported to be relieved in 80–90 percent of
patients who have the operation for chronic stable
angina. In addition, the number of heart attacks,
amount of medication needed and frequency of hospi-
talizations have been reduced. Most patients experience better exercise tolerance. However, these improvements in symptoms have not correlated with the
patient's resumption of gainful employment. Whether
or not the person returns to work depends on many
nonmedical factors (see Chapter 8).

- Angina recurs or progresses after bypass surgery in about 5 percent of the patients. Most of the new angina is associated with grafts that have not remained open or progression of the disease in the native coronary circulation. Other factors may be involved, such as failure to reduce the cholesterol levels or to control hypertension.
- The place where bypass surgery is performed counts heavily in success of the operation. It is important that there is skilled medical and technical support, as well as an experienced surgical team. Features which the consensus committee felt to be important were facilities for expertly performed angiography, appropriate laboratory and blood-banking facilities, competent anesthesiologists, the use of optimal techniques to preserve the heart muscle during surgery, a suitable intensive-care unit with competent personnel and equipment.
- Patients with chronic stable angina and normal or only moderately impaired left ventricles should expect a hospital mortality rate of no more than 4 percent. A rate of less than 1 percent is possible. The incidence of heart attack induced by surgery may be approximately 5 percent.
- For patients with unstable angina, mortality figures and heart attacks during or soon after surgery depend on the institution's approach to managing the patient. It is felt that risks to the patient are lower if there is a longer period of stabilization before proceeding to surgery. If this is done, the rate of hospital mortality and heart attack should be similar to those of patients with chronic stable angina.
- Except for emergency operations, patients with disease of the left main coronary artery can receive bypass surgery with a risk only slightly higher than

that of patients with chronic stable angina and blockages elsewhere.
· Hospital mortality rates are higher in patients who
have ejection fractions of less than 25 percent; however, even these figures have improved, and a mortality rate of no more than 15–20 percent is generally
achievable.

The panel concluded that: "Coronary artery bypass
represents a major advance in the treatment of patients
with coronary artery disease. Evidence has been presented to support the conclusion that an improvement in
the quality of life, a decrease in myocardial ischemia, and
an increase in survival have been demonstrated after coronary artery bypass in *selected subsets* of patients."

The search for reliable information continues. The National Heart, Lung, and Blood Institute is currently engaged in a Coronary Artery Surgery Study (called CASS),
a randomized effort to compare the effect of surgery with
the effect of medical management in certain subgroups of
patients.

When the study was initiated in 1974, it had already
been accepted that coronary bypass surgery was effective
for patients with incapacitating symptoms of angina.
Therefore, these patients *were not* included in the study,
nor were patients with blockages of more than *70 percent
in the left main coronary artery.*

The groups of patients, all sixty-five or younger, being
studied are:

· those with mild stable angina and normal left ventricular function (514 patients);
· those with mild stable angina and left ventricular dysfunction, but with no symptoms of heart failure (106
patients);

· patients who have no symptoms, but who have had heart attacks more than three weeks earlier (160 patients).

All patients had to have a blockage of at least 70 percent in at least one major coronary artery and distal vessels (those beyond the blocked area) suitable for bypass surgery.

All of the patients have been classified on the basis of their risk factors, their coronary anatomy (as shown on an angiogram) and their ventricular function.

The 780 patients enrolled in the study will be analyzed for:

· length of survival;
· subsequent heart attacks;
· quality of life.

No data on this study will be released until 1983.

APPENDIX II:
NUMBERS
YOU SHOULD KNOW

BLOOD PRESSURE: Normal blood pressure is considered anything from 120/80 to 140/90. However, readings lower than 120/80 (for instance, 110/70) are considered by many to be healthier. Systolic pressure of 140 to 159 is considered borderline as is diastolic pressure between 90 and 94. Systolic pressure greater than 160 or diastolic pressure higher than 95 is high.

CHOLESTEROL LEVEL: Cholesterol levels from 160 to 300 have been called normal. However, the American Heart Association feels that 200 or under is advisable. Some physicians even recommend cholesterol levels of 160 or 170.

EJECTION FRACTION: This figure, which is highly predictive of the health of the left ventricle of the heart, reflects the pumping capacity of the heart. Normal ejection fraction is 50 . . . anything higher is better, lower is worse.

HEART RATE: Resting heart rate varies from 60 to 100 beats a minute. In infants, the resting heart rate is higher —up to 130 beats a minute. Persons physically fit (such as athletes) may have lower resting heart rates. Persons under stress or participating in vigorous exercise will have higher rates.

HIGH DENSITY LIPOPROTEINS: These are the lipoproteins that are thought to be protective against coronary artery disease. Levels in males range from 35 to 60, with the mean level being 45. In women, levels range from 50 to 60, with 55 being the mean. Levels above these are considered more protective against coronary artery disease.

TRIGLYCERIDES: A blood lipid which may have some relationship to coronary artery disease, but which is yet unproven. Triglycerides normally range from 50 to 200.

☰ REFERENCES

Chapter One

American Heart Association. *The Heartbook.* New York: E. P. Dutton, 1980.

Benson, H. *The Relaxation Response.* New York: William Morrow & Co., 1975.

Brams, W.A. *Managing Your Coronary.* Published by American National Bank and Trust Co. of Chicago, 1974.

Brest, A.N. et al. *Unresolved Issues in Hypertension.* Philadelphia: Jefferson Medical College.

Chaitman, B.R. "Clinical Factors Relating to High Risk Coronary Disease in CASS." Presented at 53rd Annual Scientific Sessions, American Heart Association, November 1980, at Miami Beach, Florida.

"Cholesterol Counts," *Newsweek,* Jan. 19, 1980.

"Clue in Blood to End Cholesterol Disease," *Miami Herald,* Aug. 29, 1976.

Coronary Risk Handbook. Published by American Heart Association.

DeBakey, M., and Gotto, A: *The Living Heart.* New York: Grosset & Dunlap Co., Charter Books, 1977.

Fisher, A. *The Healthy Heart.* Library of Health. New York: Time-Life Books, 1980.

Friedman, M., and Rosenman, R. "Association of Specific Overt Behavior Pattern with Blood and Cardiovascular Findings," *Journal of the American Medical Association* 179: 1286, 1959.

Glueck, C.J. "Identification of High Risk Children." Presented at 53rd Annual Scientific Sessions, American Heart Association, November 1980, at Miami Beach, Florida.

"Good Cholesterol," *Philadelphia Daily News,* Nov. 13, 1980.

Gruchow, H.W. Presented at 53rd Annual Scientific Sessions, American Heart Association, November 1980, at Miami Beach, Florida.

Heiss, G. et al. "Good Cholesterol." Presented at 53rd Annual Scientific Sessions, American Heart Association, November 1980, at Miami Beach, Florida.

High Blood Pressure. Published by American Heart Association, 1974.

Kannel, W.B. "Oral Contraceptive Hypertension and Thromboembolism," *International Journal of Gynecology and Obstetrics* 16:466–472, 1979.

Kannel, W.B., and Dawber, T.R. "Hypertension As an Ingredient of a Cardiovascular Risk Profile," *Br. J. Hosp. Med.* 2:508, 1974.

Kannel, W.B. et al. American Heart Association, "Report of Ad Hoc Committee on Cigarette Smoking and Cardiovascular Diseases for Health Professionals," June 1, 1977.

————. "Perspectives on Systolic Hypertension, The Framingham Study," *Circulation* 61, No. 6, June 1980.

Levy, R.I. "HDFP—Implications for Health Research and National Health Care." Presented at 53rd Annual Scientific Sessions, American Heart Association, November 1980, at Miami Beach, Florida.

Morris, J.N. et al. "Vigorous Exercise in Leisure-Time: Protection Against Coronary Heart Disease." *Lancet* 2:1207–1210, Dec. 6, 1980.

Motulsky, A.G. "Atherosclerosis: Searching for the Genetic 'Tag.'" Research Report 4, American Heart Association's Seventh Science Writers' Forum, January 1980, at St. Petersburg, Florida.

1980 Report of the Joint National Committee on Detection, Evaluation, and Treatment of High Blood Pressure. Approved by National High Blood Pressure Coordinating Committee.

Olson, R.E. et al. "Toward Healthful Diets." National Research Council's Food and Nutrition Board. St. Louis University School of Medicine.

Roberts, W.C., and Waller, B.F. "Ninety-year-olds Have Conquered Coronary Heart Disease." Presented at 53rd Annual Scientific Sessions, American Heart Association, November 1980, at Miami Beach, Florida.

Shekelle, R: Diet, "Serum Cholesterol and Death from Coronary Heart Disease: The Western Electric Study," *New England Journal of Medicine* 304:65–70, Jan. 8, 1981.

Williams, R.R. "Family Roots Are an Obvious Predictor of Heart Attack Risk." Research Report 4, American Heart Association's Seventh Science Writers' Forum, January 1980, at St. Petersburg, Florida.

Zulokar, J. et al. "Leukocyte Count, Smoking and Myocardial Infarction." *New England Journal of Medicine* 304:465, Feb. 19, 1981.

Chapter Two

Garrett, H.E. et al: "Aortocoronary Bypass with Saphenous Vein Graft." *The Journal of the American Medical Association* 223:792–794, Feb. 12, 1981.

Loop, F.D. et al. "The Efficacy of Coronary Artery Surgery." *American Heart Journal* 101: 86–96, January 1981.

Manley, J.C. et al. "Ten Year Experience with the Internal Mammary Artery As a Coronary Bypass Graft," *The American Journal of Cardiology* 47:485, February 1981.

Wertenbaker, L. *To Mend the Heart.* New York: Viking Press, 1980.

Chapter Three

American Heart Association: "Computer Method Produces New Insights into Spasm and Narrowing of Arteries," *Cardiovascular Research Report,* 8:2, Spring 1981.

Benrey, J. et al. "Negative Treadmill Exercise Test Result with Subsequent Myocardial Infarction and Coronary Artery Bypass: Case Report," *Cardiovascular Diseases, Bulletin of the Texas Heart Institute* 5:391, December 1978.

Brody, J.E. "Personal Health," *The New York Times,* Dec. 13, 1978.

Coronary Risk Handbook. Published by American Heart Association, Committee on Reduction of Risk of Heart Attack and Stroke, 1973.

Dranov, P. "Stress Tests: Getting to the Heart of the Controversy," *Family Weekly* Dec. 2, 1979.

Epstein, S.E.: "Implications of Probability Analysis on the Strategy Employed for the Noninvasive Detection of Coronary Artery Disease: Role of Single or Combined Use of Exercise ECG Testing, Radionuclide Cineangiography and Myocardial Perfusion Imaging," *American Journal of Cardiology* 46:491–99, 1980.

Forrester, J., and Diamond, G. "How to Screen for Coronary Artery Disease." Presented at 53rd Annual Scientific Sessions, American Heart Association, November 1980, at Miami Beach, Florida.

Harvard Medical School Health Letter: "A Leisurely Look at Stress," October 1979.

Hollenberg, M. "New Computerized Scoring System Improves Accuracy of Treadmill Exercising Testing." Presented at 53rd Annual Scientific Sessions, American Heart Association, November 1980, at Miami Beach, Florida.

James, T.N. "Presidential Address." Presented at 53rd Annual Scientific Sessions, American Heart Association, November 1980, at Miami Beach, Florida.

Maranhao, V. "Catheterization Procedures." Deborah Heart and Lung Center, Catheterization Laboratory.

McIntosh, H.D., and Garcia, J.A. "First Decade of Aortocoronary Bypass Grafting, 1967–1977," *Circulation* 57:405–428, March 1978.

Perrigo, E.S. et al. "20-Month Experience in Outpatient Cardiac Catheterization." Presented at 53rd Annual Scientific Sessions, American Heart Association, November 1980, at

Miami Beach, Florida. Abstract published *Circulation,* October 1980.

Sifford, D. "Computers Join Doctors to Care for Your Heart," *Philadelphia Inquirer,* Sept. 25, 1980.

The Center Post: Presbyterian-University of Pennsylvania Medical Center. "Gamma Camera, New Diagnostic Procedure in Cardiology Center" 5:4–5, November–December, 1978.

Chapter Four

Campeau, L. *The Place of Aorto-Coronary By-Pass Surgery in the Treatment of Ischemic Heart Disease. Atherosclerosis.* Plenum Publishing Co., 1977.

Campeau, L. et al. "Left Main Coronary Artery Stenosis: The Influence of Aortocoronary Bypass Surgery on Survival," *Circulation* 57:1111–1115, 1978.

Chaitman, B.R. "Survival Patterns in Left Main Coronary Disease Subsets: Results of the CASS Study." Presented at the American Heart Association Scientific Sessions, November 19, 1980, at Miami Beach, Florida.

Conley M.J. et al. "The Prognostic Spectrum of Left Main Stenosis," *Circulation* 57:947–952, 1978.

Conti, C.R. and Christie, L.G. Jr. "Coronary Artery Bypass Surgery: A Cardiology Viewpoint," *Cardiovascular Reviews and Reports,* vol. 2, pp. 127–137, February 1981.

Conti, C.R. et al. "Unstable Angina Pectoris—NHLBI Trial: Effects of Early Non-Fatal Myocardial Infarction on Subsequent Mortality and Symptoms (abstr.)," *Circulation* 58 (suppl. II):152, 1978.

Corday, E. et al: "Medical versus Surgical Treatment of Coronary Artery Disease—1981." *Cardiovascular Reviews and Reports* 2, No. 3:281–287, March 1981.

DeBakey, M.E., and Lawrie, G.M.: "Coronary Arterial Bypass: Current Status." Pre-publication.

Detre, K. et al. "Effect of Bypass Surgery on Survival in Patients in Low and High Risk Subgroups Delineated by the Use of Simple Clinical Variables." *Circulation* 63:1329–1338, June 1981.

Epstein, S.E. et al. "Strategy for Evaluation and Surgical Treatment of the Asymptomatic or Mildly Symptomatic Patient with Coronary Artery Disease," *American Journal of Cardiology* 43:1015–1025, May 1979.

Favaloro, R.G. "Direct Myocardial Revascularization: A Ten-Year Journey," *American Journal of Cardiology* 43:109, January 1979.

Gazes, P.C. et al. "Pre-infarction (unstable) Angina—A Prospective Study—Ten-Year Follow-up Prognostic Significance of Electrocardiographic Changes," *Circulation* 48:331, 1973.

Gould, K.L., and Lipscomb, K. "Effects of Coronary Stenosis on Coronary Flow Reserve and Resistance," *American Journal of Cardiology* 34:48, 1974.

Grondin, C.M. et al. "Prophylactic Coronary Artery Grafting in Patients with Few or No Symptoms," *Annals of Thoracic Surgery* 28:113–118, August 1979.

Hughes, D.A. et al. *Coronary Artery Surgery in the Young Adult. Coronary Artery Medicine and Surgery: Concepts and Controversies.* New York: Appleton-Century-Crofts, 1975, pp. 804–808.

Hurst, J.W. et al. "Value of Coronary Bypass Surgery," *American Journal of Cardiology* 42:308–329, August 1978.

Johnson, W.D. "Late Results in Coronary Vein Grafts," *Cardiovascular Disease*, 1974.

————. "Diffuse Coronary Artery Disease: Is It a Contra-Indication for Surgery?" Presented at International Symposium, Coronary Heart Surgery: A Rehabilitation Measure, March 1978, at Bad Krozingen, West Germany.

Kouchoukos, N.T. et al. "Coronary Bypass Surgery: Analysis of Factors Affecting Hospital Mortality," *Circulation* 62 (suppl. I) 1–84, 1980.

Lim, J.S. et al. "Left Main Coronary Arterial Obstruction: Long-term follow-up of 141 non-surgical cases," *American Journal of Cardiology* 36:131–135, 1975.

Loop, F.D. et al. "The Efficacy of Coronary Artery Surgery." *American Heart Journal* 101: 86–96, January 1981.

Maseri, A. "Coronary Artery Spasm." Delivered at 25th Annual James B. Herrick Memorial Lecture before Chicago Heart Association, February 1981, at Chicago, Illinois.

Mason, D.T. et al. *The Prevention of Myocardial Infarction by Coronary Bypass Surgery. The Heart Update II.* Hurst, J.W., ed. New York: McGraw-Hill Book Co., 1980, p. 103.

McIntosh, H.D., and Garcia, J.A. "The First Decade of Aortocoronary Bypass Grafting, 1967–1977," *Circulation* 57:405, March 1978.

McNeer, J.F. et al. "The Nature of Treatment Selection in Coronary Artery Disease," *Circulation* XLIX:606–614, April 1974.

Meyer, J. et al. "Coronary Artery Bypass in Patients Over 70 Years of Age: Indications and Results," *American Journal of Cardiology* 36:342–345, September 1975.

Miller, D.W. Jr. et al. "The Practice of Coronary Artery Bypass Surgery in 1980." Presented at American Heart Association Scientific Sessions, November 1980, at Miami Beach, Florida.

Murphy, M.L. et al. "Treatment of Chronic Stable Angina; a preliminary report of survival data of the randomized Veterans Administration Cooperative Study," *New England Journal of Medicine* 297:621–627, 1977.

Podrid, P.J. et al. "Prognosis of Medically Treated Patients with Coronary-Artery Disease with Profound ST-Segment Depression During Exercise Testing," *New England Journal of Medicine* 305:1111–16, Nov. 5, 1981.

Proudfit, W.L. et al. "Natural History of Obstructive Coronary Artery Disease: 10-year study of 601 non-surgical cases," *Prog. Cardiovascular Disease* 21:53, 1978.

Rosati, R.A. et al. "A New Information System for Medical Practice," *Archives of Internal Medicine* 135:1017–1024, August 1975.

———. "Does Coronary Surgery Prolong Life in Comparison with Medical Management?" *Postgraduate Medical Journal* 52:749–756, 1976.

Selden, R. et al. "Medical versus Surgical Therapy for Acute Coronary Insufficiency," *New England Journal of Medicine* 293:1329, 1975.

Sheldon, W.C. et al. "Bypass Graft Surgery for Coronary Artery Disease: a 10–13 year follow-up study of 741 patients," *American Journal of Cardiology.* In press.

———. "Surgical Treatment of Coronary Artery Disease," *Prog. Cardiovascular Dis.* 18:240–252, 1975.

Sung, R.J. et al. "Left Main Coronary Artery Obstruction. Follow-up of Thirty Patients With and Without Surgery." *Circulation* 51 and 52 (suppl. I): 1–112, 1975.

Vakil, R.J. "Pre-infarction Syndrome-Management and Follow-Up," *American Journal of Cardiology* 14:55, 1964.

Wertenbaker, L. *To Mend the Heart.* New York: Viking Press, 1980.

Chapter Five

Al-Bassam, M.S. et al. "Evaluation of Risk Factors and Follow-Up in Women Following Coronary Artery Bypass," *Cardiovascular Diseases, Bulletin of the Texas Heart Institute* 2:391, 1975.

Alderman, E.L. et al. "Evaluation of Enzyme Testing for the Detection of Myocardial Infarction Following Direct Coronary Surgery," *Circulation* 48:135, 1973.

Aldridge, H.E., and Trimble, A.S. "Progression of Proximal Coronary Artery Lesions to Total Occlusion After Aortocoronary Saphenous Vein Bypass Grafting," *Journal of Thoracic Cardiovascular Surgery* 62:7, 1971.

American Heart Association: *Inside the Cardiac Care Unit. A Guide for the Patient and Family.*

Aronow, W.S., and Stemmer, E.A. "Two-Year Follow-Up of Angina Pectoris: Medical or Surgical Therapy," *Ann. Intern. Med.* 82:208, 1975.

Assad-Morell, J.L. et al. "Relation of Intraoperative or Early Postoperative Transmural Myocardial Infarction to Patency of Aortocoronary Bypass Grafts and to Diseased Ungrafted Coronary Arteries," *American Journal of Cardiology* 35:767, 1975.

Benchimol, A. et al. "Electrovectorcardiographic Changes After Proximal Right Coronary Artery Venous Bypass Graft and Distal Gas Endarterectomy," *American Journal of Cardiology* 30:466, 1972.

Bolooki, H., and Vargas, A. "Myocardial Revascularization After Acute Myocardial Infarction," *Arch. Surg.* 111:1216, 1976.

Blumlein, S.L. et al. "Preoperative Risk Factors and Aortocoronary Bypass Graft Patency," *Journal of Thoracic Cardiovascular Surgery* 72:778, 1976.

Bourassa, M.G. et al. "Progression of Coronary Disease Five to Seven Years After Aortocoronary Bypass Surgery." Delivered at the 3rd International Symposium, Coronary Heart Disease, February 1978, at Frankfurt, Germany.

————. "Progression of Obstructive Coronary Artery Disease 5 to 7 Years After Aortocoronary Bypass Surgery," *Circulation* 57 and 58 (suppl. I):1–100, 1978.

Breuer, A.C. et al. "Brain and Nerve Injury Associated with Coronary Bypass Surgery, Prospective Study of 421 Cases." Delivered at the 53rd Annual Scientific Sessions, American Heart Association, November 1980, at Miami Beach, Florida.

Campeau, L. et al. "Loss of the Improvement of Angina Between 1 and 7 Years After Aortocoronary Bypass Surgery." Cardiovascular Surgery, supp. 1, *Circulation* 60:I-1–5, 1978.

————. "Recurrence of Angina After Coronary Bypass Surgery," *The Journal of Cardiovascular Medicine* 6, 1981.

Cooley, D.A. "Aortocoronary Artery Bypass: Present Indications, Risk Factors and Long-term Survival." Presented at World Congress on Vascular Diseases, 1976, at Bombay, India.

――――. "Direct Myocardial Revascularization: Experience with 9,364 Operations," *Thorax* 33:411, August 1978.

Cooley, D.A. et al. "Aortocoronary Saphenous Vein Bypass," *Annals of Thoracic Surgery* 16:380, October 1973.

Cooley, D.A., and Wormuth, C.E. "Direct Coronary Surgery," *AORN Journal* 21:789, April 1975.

Cosgrove, D.M. et al. "Blood Conservation During Myocardial Revascularization," *Ann. Thorac. Surg.* 28:184, 1979.

Crawford, E.S. et al. "Operative Risk in Patients with Previous Coronary Artery Bypass," *Ann. Thorac. Surg.* 26:215, 1978.

Douglas, J.S., Jr., et al. "Reduced Efficacy of Coronary Bypass Surgery in Women." Presented at 53rd Scientific Sessions, American Heart Association, November 1980.

Du Cailar, C. et al. "Risks and Benefits of Aortocoronary Bypass Surgery in Patients Aged 65 Years or More," *CMA Journal* 122:771–774, Apr. 5, 1980.

Dunkman, W.B. et al. "Medical Perspectives in Coronary Artery Surgery—A Caveat," *Ann. Intern. Med.* 81:817, 1974.

Epstein, S.E.: "Implications of Probability Analysis on the Strategy Employed for the Noninvasive Detection of Coronary Artery Disease: Role of Single or Combined Use of Exercise ECG Testing, Radionuclide Cineangiography and Myocardial Perfusion Imaging," *American Journal of Cardiology* 46:491–99, 1980.

Espinoza, J. et al. "New Q-Waves After Coronary Artery Bypass Surgery for Angina Pectoris," *American Journal of Cardiology* 33:221, 1974.

Favaloro, R.G. "Direct Myocardial Revascularization: A Ten-Year Journey," *American Journal of Cardiology* 43:109, January 1979.

Fennel, W. et al. "Significance of Appearance of Serum CPK-MB Following Bypass Surgery," *Clinical Research* 25:221A, 1977.

Flemma, R.J. et al. "Factors Predictive of Perioperative Myocardial Infarction During Coronary Operations," *Annals of Thoracic Surgery* 21:215, 1976.

Frommer, P. et al. "Multivariate Discriminant Analysis of the Clinical and Angiographic Predictors of Operative Mortality from the Collaborative Study in Coronary Artery Surgery (CASS)." Delivered at the 53rd Annual Scientific Sessions, American Heart Association, November 1980, at Miami Beach, Florida.

Gott, V.L. "Outlook for Patients After Coronary Artery Revascularization," *American Journal of Cardiology* 33:431, 1974.

Griffith, L.S.C. et al. "Changes in Intrinsic Coronary Circulation and Segmental Ventricular Motion After Saphenous Vein Coronary Bypass Graft Surgery," *New England Journal of Medicine* 288:589, 1973.

Grondin, P. et al. "Preoperative Left Ventricular Ejection Fraction and Survival After Coronary Artery Surgery," *The Canadian Journal of Surgery,* November 1976.

Gunstenson, J. et al. "Evolving Indications for Preoperative Intraaortic Balloon Pump Assistance," *Annals of Thoracic Surgery* 22:535, 1976.

Hamby, R.I. et al. "Left Ventricular Hemodynamics and Contractible Pattern After Aortocoronary Bypass Surgery—Factors Affecting Reversibility of Abnormal Left Ventricular Function," *American Heart Journal* 88:149, 1974.

Hammermeister, K.E. et al. "Effect of Aortocoronary Saphenous Vein Bypass Grafting on Death and Sudden Death," *American Journal of Cardiology* 39:925, 1977.

———. "Evidence from a Nonrandomized Study That Coronary Surgery Prolongs Survival in Patients with Two-Vessel Coronary Disease," *Circulation* 59:430, 1979.

———. "Predictors of Surgical Mortality in Patients Undergoing Direct Myocardial Revascularization," *Circulation Supp. II.* 50:112–115, 1974.

———. "Variables Predictive of Survival in Patients with Coronary Disease," *Circulation* 59:421–430, March 1979.

Harlan, B.J. et al. "Treatment of Severe Coronary Artery Disease with Quadruple and Quintuple Saphenous Vein Grafts," *Chest* 69:29, January 1976.

Harris, P.J. et al. "Nonfatal Myocardial Infarction in Medically Treated Patients with Coronary Artery Disease," *American Journal of Cardiology* 46:973, December 1980.

———. "Survival in Medically Treated Coronary Artery Disease," *Circulation* 60:1259, 1979.

Hoffmann, R.G. et al. "The Probability of Surviving Coronary Bypass Surgery," *Journal of American Medical Association* 243:1341, Apr. 4, 1980.

"In His Own Words: One Out of Every Three Operations Is Unwise, Says Surgeon George Crile," *People* magazine, Mar. 19, 1979.

Itscoitz, S.B. et al. "Saphenous Vein Bypass Grafts: Long-term Patency and Effect on the Native Coronary Circulation," *American Journal of Cardiology* 36:745, 1975.

Johnson, W.D. "Diffuse Coronary Artery Disease: Is It a Contraindication for Surgery?" Presented at International Symposium, Coronary Heart Surgery: A Rehabilitation Measure, March 1978, at Bad Krozingen, West Germany.

Johnson, W.D. et al. "Six Years' Experience Using Four to Seven Bypass Grafts Per Patient." Presented at the 12th Annual Meeting of the Society of Thoracic Surgeons, January 1976, at Washington, D.C.

Kouchoukos, N.T. et al. "An Appraisal of Coronary Bypass Grafting," *Circulation* 50:11, 1974.

———. "Coronary Bypass Surgery: Analysis of Factors Affecting Hospital Mortality," *Circulation* 62, suppl. I:1–84, 1980.

Lear, M.W. *Heartsounds.* New York: Simon and Schuster, 1980.

Logue, B. SBII, and Douglas, J.S., Jr. "A Practical Approach to Coronary Artery Disease with Special Reference to Coronary Artery Bypass Surgery," *Current Prob. Cardio.* 1:5, 1976.

Loop, F.D. et al. "Atherosclerosis of the Left Main Coronary Artery: Five-Year Results of Surgical Treatment," *American Journal of Cardiology* 44:195, 1979.

———. "The Efficacy of Coronary Artery Surgery." *American Heart Journal* 101: 86–96, January 1981.

———. "An 11-Year Evolution of Coronary Arterial Surgery (1967–1978)," *Ann. Surg.* 190:444, 1979.

Manley, J.C. et al. "The 'Bad' Left Ventricle," *Journal of Thoracic Cardiovascular Surgery* 72:841, 1976.

Mason, D.T. "Improved Longevity Due to Reduction of Sudden Death by Aortocoronary Bypass in Coronary Atherosclerosis," *American Journal of Cardiology* 39:919, 1977.

Mathur, V.S. "Prospective Randomized Study of the Surgical Therapy of Stable Angina," *Cardiovascular Clin.* 8(2):131, 1977.

Maurer, B.J. et al. "Changes in Grafted and Nongrafted Coronary Arteries Following Saphenous Vein Bypass Grafting," *Circulation* 50:293, 1974.

McIntosh, H.D. et al. "Indications for Saphenous Vein Aortocoronary Bypass Surgery," *Athero. Rev.* 1:183, 1976.

McIntosh, H.D., and Garcia, J.A. "The First Decade of Aortocoronary Bypass Grafting, 1967–1977," *Circulation* 57:405, March 1978.

Meyer, J. et al. "The Value of Moderate Hypothermia During Anoxic Cardiac Arrest for Coronary Artery Surgery," *Journal of Cardiovascular Surgery* 16:465, September–October 1975.

Miller, D.W., Jr. "Bypass Surgery for Coronary Heart Disease." University of Washington School of Medicine.

Miller, D.W., Jr., et al. "The Practice of Coronary Artery Bypass Surgery in 1980." Presented at 53rd Scientific Sessions, American Heart Association, November 1980, at Miami Beach, Florida.

Millman, M. "Bypass Surgery: Does Anybody Need It But the Surgeons?" *New West*, Sept. 13, 1976.

Morton, B.C. et al. "Myocardial Infarction: Coronary Artery Surgery," *Circulation* 51, 52 (suppl.): I–198, 1975.

Mundth, E.D., and Austen, W.G. "Surgical Measures for Coronary Heart Disease," *New England Journal of Medicine* 293:13, 75–124, 1975.

Murphy, M.L. et al. "Treatment of Chronic Stable Angina. A Preliminary Report of Survival Data of the Randomized Veterans Administration Cooperative Study," *New England Journal of Medicine* 297:621, 1977.

Oberman, A. et al. "Survival Following Perioperative Myocardial Infarction. Presented at 53rd Scientific Sessions, American Heart Association, November 1980, at Miami Beach, Florida.

Oglietti, J. et al. "Myocardial Revascularization." *The Journal of Thoracic and Cardiovascular Surgery* 71:736, May 1976.

Oldham, H.N., Jr., et al. "Intraoperative Detection of Myocardial Damage During Coronary Artery Surgery by Plasma Creatine Phosphokinase Isoenzyme Analysis," *Surgery* 74:917, 1973.

Phillips, D.F. et al. "Perioperative Myocardial Infarction: Angiographic Correlations," *American Journal of Cardiology* 39:269, 1977.

Proudfit, W.L. et al. "Natural History of Obstructive Coronary Artery Disease: 10-Year Study of 601 Nonsurgical Cases," *Prog. Cardiovasc. Dis.* 21:53, 1978.

Reeves, T.J. et al. "Natural History of Angina Pectoris," *American Journal of Cardiology* 33:423, 1974.

Reul, G.J. et al. "Aortocoronary Artery Bypass," *Archives of Surgery* 11:414–418, April 1976.

Sandiford, F.M. et al. "The Aortocoronary Bypass Operation: Myth and Reality. An Overview Based on 10,000 Operations at the Texas Heart Institute," *International Surgery* 63, 1978.

Scannell, J.G. et al. "Criteria for Surgery: Optimal Resources for Cardiac Surgery," *Circulation* 44:A221, 1971.

Schrank, J.P. et al. "The Incidence and Clinical Significance of ECG—VCG Changes of Myocardial Infarction Following Aortocoronary Saphenous Vein Bypass Surgery," *American Heart Journal* 87:46, 1974.

Spencer, F.C. et al. "Significance of Air Embolism During Cardiopulmonary Bypass," *Journal of Thoracic Cardiovascular Surgery* 49:615, 1965.

Sternberg, L. et al. "Significance of New Q-Waves After Aortocoronary Bypass Surgery. Correlation with Changes in Ventricular Wall Motion," *Circulation* 52:1037, 1975.

Stoney, W.S. et al. "Unexpected Death Following Aortocoronary Bypass," *Annals of Thoracic Surgery* 21:528, 1976.

Walen, R.E. et al. "The Natural History of Coronary Artery Disease: An Update on Surgical and Medical Management," *Trans. Am. Clin. Climatol. Assoc.* 89:19, 1977.

Wukasch, D.C. et al. "Reoperation Following Direct Myocardial Revascularization," *Cardiovascular Surgery supp. 2, Circulation* 56:I-3-7, 1977.

————. "Reoperation Following Direct Myocardial Revascularization." Presented at the 49th Annual Scientific Sessions, American Heart Association, November 1976, at Miami Beach, Florida.

————. "Surgical Treatment of Angina Pectoris: Current Status," *Angiology* 28:169, March 1977.

————. "Surgical vs Medical Treatment of Coronary Artery Disease: Long-Term Survival," *Vascular Surgery* 10, no. 5:300, November–December 1976.

Chapter Six

Baber, N.S. et al. "Multicentre Post-Infarction Trial of Propranolol in 49 Hospitals in the United Kingdom, Italy, and Yugoslavia," *British Medical Journal* 44:96–100, 1979.

Barndt, R. et al. "Regression and Progression of Early Atherosclerosis in Treated Hyperlipidemic Patients," *Annals of Internal Medicine* 86:139–146, 1977.

Bonow, R.O. et al. "Effects of Verapamil Alone and Combined with Propranolol on Left Ventricular Systolic Function in Patients with Coronary Artery Disease." Presented at 53rd Scientific Sessions, American Heart Association, November 1980, at Miami Beach, Florida.

Grady, D. "Stopping a Heart Attack," *Discover* January 1981.

Harris, P.J. et al. "Outcome in Medically Treated Coronary Artery Disease—Ischemic Events: Non-fatal Infarction and Death," *Circulation* 62:718–726, 1980.

————. "Survival in Medically Treated Coronary Artery Disease," *Circulation* 60:1259–69, December 1979.

Hurst, J.W. *Drugs Used in the Treatment of Coronary Atherosclerotic Heart Disease. In Update II: The Heart,* Hurst, J.W., ed. New York: McGraw-Hill, 1978, pp. 1234–41.

Leon, M.B. et al. "Clinical Efficacy of Verapamil Alone and Combined with Propranolol in Treating Patients with Chronic Stable Angina Pectoris." Presented at 53rd Scientific Sessions,

American Heart Association, November 1980, at Miami Beach, Florida.

McNeer, J.F. et al. "The Nature of Treatment Selection in Coronary Artery Disease," *Circulation* XLIX:606–615, April 1974.

"Multicentre International Study: Improvement in Prognosis of Myocardial Infarction by Long-term Beta-adrenoreceptor Blockade Using Practolol," *British Medical Journal* 3:735–740, 1975.

Nash, D.T. et al. "The Effect of Lipid-Lowering Therapy on the Progression and Regression of Coronary Atherosclerosis." Presented at the 53rd Scientific Sessions, American Heart Association, November 1980, at Miami Beach, Florida.

Norwegian Multicenter Study Group: "Timolol—Induced Reduction in Mortality and Reinfarction in Patients Surviving Acute Myocardial Infarction. *New England Journal of Medicine* 304, Issue 14:801–807, Apr. 2, 1981.

Schroeder, J.S. "Calcium Antagonists: Use in Coronary Artery Disease. Results of Clinical Trials in Unstable Angina Pectoris." Presented at 53rd Scientific Sessions, American Heart Association, November 1980, at Miami Beach, Florida.

Chapter Seven

Anderson, A.J. et al. "Retention or Resumption of Employment After Aortocoronary Bypass Operations," *Journal of American Medical Association* 243:543–545, Feb. 8, 1980.

Barboriak, J.J. et al. "Alcohol and Coronary Arteries," *Alcoholism: Clinical and Experimental Research* 3:29–32, 1979.

———. "Coronary Artery Occlusion and Alcohol Intake," *British Heart Journal* 39:289–293, 1977.

Bierman, E.L. et al. *Diet and Coronary Heart Disease.* American Heart Association, 1978.

Blumlein, S.L. et al. "Changes in Occupation After Coronary Arteriography," *Scandinavia Journal of Rehabilitation Medicine* 9:79–83, 1977.

Dawber, T.R., and Kannel, W.B. "Current Status of Coronary Prevention. Lessons from the Framingham Study," *Preventive Medicine* 1:499–512, 1972.

Grundy, S.M. "Are Triglycerides a Risk Factor for Coronary Heart Disease?" Presented at Nutrition and Heart Disease: The 1981 Perspective, 1981, at New York City.

————. "Background Statement: The Relationship Between Low Cholesterol Levels and Cancer." Presented at Nutrition and Heart Disease: The 1981 Perspective, 1981, at New York City.

Hammermeister, K.E. et al. "Effect of Surgical Versus Medical Therapy on Return to Work in Patients with Coronary Artery Disease," *American Journal of Cardiology* 44:105–11, July 1979.

Kannel, W.B. *Risk Factors in Coronary Disease—Disease Update. CME Medicine.* John Wiley & Sons, Inc., 1979.

Kannel, W.B. et al. "Risk Factors and Coronary Disease," *American Heart Association Committee Report,* May 1980.

Kannel, W.B., and Sorlie, P. "Some Health Benefits of Physical Activity. The Framingham Study," *Archives of Internal Medicine* 139:857–861, August 1979.

Kannel, W.B., and Thom, T.J. "Implications of the Recent Decline in Cardiovascular Mortality," *Cardiovascular Medicine* 4:983–997, September 1979.

Kasl, S.V. "The Effect of Stress and Other Psychosocial Factors in the Development of Coronary Heart Disease, *Washington Public Health* 2:18.

Lasser, N.L. "What the AHA is Doing in Nutrition Programs for the Public." Presented at Nutrition and Heart Disease: The 1981 Perspective, 1981, at New York City.

Mahley, R.W. "How Lipoproteins Respond to a Fat-Rich Diet." Presented at Nutrition and Heart Disease: The 1981 Perspective, 1981, at New York City.

Oberman, A., and Kouchoukos, N.T. "Working Status of Patients Following Coronary Bypass Surgery," *American Heart Journal* 98:132–133, July 1979.

Ribakove, B.M. "Balancing the Fat Lowers the Blood Pressure," *Family Health,* November–December 1980.

Rimm, A.O. et al. "Changes in Occupation After Aortocoronary Vein By-Pass Operation," *Journal of the American Medical Association* 236:361–364, 1976.

Tall, A.R. "How the Body Responds to a Fat-Rich Meal." Presented at Nutrition and Heart Disease: The 1981 Perspective, 1981, at New York City.

Williams, R.B., Jr. *Behavioral Factors in Cardiovascular Disease: An Update.* In Update: The Heart, Hurst, J.W. ed. vol. V. New York: McGraw-Hill, 1981.

Williams, R.B., Jr., et al. "A 'Prognostigram' Seeks to Predict Who'll Get Relief from Heart Pain." Delivered at 53rd Annual Scientific Sessions, American Heart Association, November 1980, at Miami Beach, Florida.

Chapter Eight

Bentivoglio, L.G. "Bypassing the Bypass with Percutaneous Transluminal Coronary Angioplasty," *American Journal of Cardiology* 43:866–67, April 1979.

————. "Percutaneous Transluminal Coronary Angioplasty," *Annals of Internal Medicine* 90:850–51, May 1979.

Buchwald, H. "Partial Ileal Bypass Operation in the Management of the Hyperlipidemias," *Surg. Gynecol. Obstet.* 124:1231, 1967.

Buchwald, H. et al. "Surgical Treatment of Hyperlipidemia," *Circulation* XLIX suppl. I:I–1 to I–37, 1974.

Clarke, N.E. et al. *American Journal of Medical Science* 230:654, 1956.

Dorée, C. "The Occurrence and Distribution of Cholesterol and Allied Bodies in the Animal Kingdom." *Biochem. J.,* 4:72, 1909.

Dotter, C.T., and Judkins, M.P. "Transluminal Treatment of Arteriosclerotic Obstruction," *Circulation* 30:662–675, 1964.

Gordon, G.B., and Vance, R.B. *EDTA Chelation Therapy for Arteriosclerosis: History and Mechanisms of Action.* New York: Insight Publishing Co., 1976.

Grüntzig, A.R. "Transluminal Dilatation of Coronary Artery Stenosis," *Lancet* I:263, 1978.

Grüntzig, A. et al. "Coronary Percutaneous Transluminal Angioplasty: Preliminary Results," *Circulation* 58:56, 1978.

Heydenreich, L.H. *Leonardo da Vinci,* vol. I and II. New York and Basel: Macmillan-Holbein, 1954.

Hochman, G. "Heart Bypass Surgery: Is It Worth the Risk?" *The Philadelphia Inquirer, Today Magazine.* Aug. 5, 1979.

Holmes, W.L. et al. *Hyperlipidemia-Atherosclerosis Study.* Lankenau Hospital, Philadelphia, Pa.

Isaacs, B. "Can This New Diet Prevent Heart Attacks?" *New York Magazine,* Nov. 8, 1976.

Jukes, C. "Rinse Breakfast," *Prevention Magazine,* June 1975.

Kanemoto, N. "Non-Invasive Assessment of Left Ventricular Performance Following Transluminal Coronary Angioplasty." Presented at 53rd Scientific Sessions, American Heart Association, November 1980.

Kent, KM. "PTCA Termed 'Relatively Safe' By Cooperative Study Group." Presented at 53rd Scientific Sessions, American Heart Association, November 1980.

Levy, R.I. et al. "Percutaneous Transluminal Coronary Angioplasty," *New England Journal of Medicine* 301:101–103, July 12, 1979.

Mock, M.B. et al. The National Heart, Lung, and Blood Institute Percutaneous Transluminal Coronary Angioplasty Registry: The First 1116 Cases (prior to publication).

Moore, R.B. et al. "The Effect of Partial Ileal Bypass on Plasma Lipoproteins," *Circulation* 62, No. 3:469–476, 1980.

Passwater, R. *Supernutrition for Healthy Hearts.* New York: Dial Press, 1977.

Pritikin, N. et al. "Evaluation of Inpatient Program. An Analysis of 893 Patients," *Preventive Medicine,* Summer 1981.

Report by a Research Committee of the Scottish Society of Physicians: "Ischemic Heart Disease: A Secondary Prevention Trial Using Clofibrate," *Brit. Med.* W:775, 1971.

Stertzer, S.H. et al. "Dilatation of Obstructed Coronaries by Percutaneous Transluminal Angioplasty," *Journal of Cardiovascular Medicine*, 5:1059–1064 December 1980.

———. "Evaluation of Transluminal Coronary Angioplasty in Left Main Coronary Artery Stenosis," *American Journal of Cardiology* 47:396, February 1981.

———. "Transluminal Coronary Artery Dilatation," *Practical Cardiology* 5, No. 3:25, March 1979.

Summary Statement: POSCH Project. Department of Health, Education and Welfare.

"Symposium on Atromid: Proceedings of a Conference in Buxton (England), June 5, 1965," *J. Atheroscler.* Res. 3:341, 1965.

The Pritikin Diet. Pritikin Longevity Center, Santa Monica, California.

U.S. Dept. of Health, Education and Welfare: "Proceedings of the Workshop on Percutaneous Transluminal Coronary Angioplasty," June 15–16, 1979. Published March 1980.

Appendix

Braunwald, E. "Coronary-Artery Surgery at the Crossroads," *New England Journal of Medicine* 297:661–63, Sept. 22, 1977.

Bruce, R.A. et al. "Noninvasive Screening Criteria for Enhanced 4-Year Survival After Aortocoronary Bypass Surgery," *Circulation* 60:638–46, 1979.

Bruschke, A. et al. "Progress Study of 590 Consecutive Nonsurgical Cases of Coronary Disease Followed Five to Nine Years," *Circulation* 47:1147–53, 1973.

_____. "Progress Study of 590 Consecutive Nonsurgical Cases of Coronary Disease Followed Five to Nine Years. II Ventriculographic and Other Correlations," *Circulation* 47:1154–63, 1973.

Campeau, L. et al. "Surgical Treatment of Coronary Artery Disease," *Medicine North America* 4:438–46, September 1980.

Chaitman, B.R. "Survival Patterns in Left Main Coronary Disease Subsets: Results of the CASS Study." From the Montreal Heart Institute and Participating CASS Sites. Presented at the 53rd Annual Scientific Sessions, American Heart Association, 1980, at Miami Beach, Florida.

Chalmers, T.C. et al. "In Defense of the VA Randomized Control Trial of Coronary Artery Surgery," *Clinical Res.* 26:230–35, 1978.

Cooley, D.A. et al. "Direct Myocardial Revascularization: Experience with 9,364 Operations," *Thorax* 33:411–17, August 1978.

Cooperative Unstable Angina Study Group: Unstable Angina Pectoris: National Cooperative Study Group to Compare Medical and Surgical Therapy I. "A Report of Protocol and Patient Population," *American Journal of Cardiology* 37:896–902, 1976.

Cooperative Unstable Angina Study Group: Unstable Angina Pectoris: National Cooperative Study Group to Compare Surgical and Medical Therapy II. "In-Hospital Experience and Initial Follow-up Results in Patients with One, Two and Three Vessel Disease," *American Journal of Cardiology* 42:839–48, 1978.

Cooperative Unstable Angina Study Group: National Cooperative Study Group to Compare Surgical and Medical Therapy III. "Results in Patients with ST Segment Elevation During Pain," *American Journal of Cardiology* 45:819–24, April 1980.

DeBakey, M.E., and Lawrie, G.M. "Response to Commentary of Hultgren et al on 'Aortocoronary-Artery-Bypass': Assessment After 13 Years," *The Journal of the American Medical Association* 241:2393–95, June 1, 1979.

DeRouen, T.A. et al. "Comparisons of the Effects on Survival After Coronary Artery Surgery in Subgroups of Patients from the Seattle Heart Watch," *Circulation* 63:537–45, 1981.

Epstein, S.E. et al. "Strategy for Evaluation and Surgical Treatment of the Asymptomatic or Mildly Symptomatic Patient with Coronary Artery Disease," *American Journal of Cardiology* 43:1015–25, May 1979.

European Cooperative Study. "Coronary-Artery Bypass Surgery in Stable Angina Pectoris: Second Interim Report." *Lancet* 491–495, September 1980.

Frye, R.L. et al. National Institutes of Health Consensus Development Conference Statement. "Coronary Artery Bypass Surgery: Scientific and Clinical Aspects." Developed at the National Institutes of Health, December 3–5, 1980.

Gaasch, W.H. et al. "Surgical Management of Prinzmetal's Variant Angina," *Chest* 66:614–21, 1974.

Hall, R.J. et al. "Long-Term Results of Coronary Artery Bypass," *Cardiovascular Diseases, Bulletin of the Texas Heart Institute* 3:22–31, 1976.

Hammermeister, K.E. et al. "Effect of Aortocoronary Saphenous Vein Bypass Grafting on Death and Sudden Death," *American Journal of Cardiology* 39:925–34, May 1977.

_____. "Effect of Coronary Surgery on Survival in Asymptomatic and Minimally Symptomatic Patients. Cardiovascular Surgery, 1979," Suppl. to *Circulation* 62:I-98–102, August 1980.

_____. "Effect of Saphenous Vein Bypass Grafting on Myocardial Infarction and Sudden Cardiac Death." International Congress Series 491, May 8, 1979, at Florence International Meeting on Myocardial Infarction.

_____. "Evidence from a Nonrandomized Study That Coronary Surgery Prolongs Survival in Patients with Two-Vessel Coronary Disease," *Circulation* 59:430–35, 1979.

Harris, P.J. et al. "Outcome in Medically Treated Coronary Artery Disease. Ischemic Events: Nonfatal Infarction and Death," *Circulation* 62:718–26, October 1980.

_____. "Survival in Medically Treated Coronary Artery Disease," *Circulation* 60:1259–69, December 1979.

Johnson, W.D., and Shore, R.T. "Coronary Bypass Surgery: Early and Long-Term Results." Advances in the Management of Clinical Heart Diseases (Monograph Series—Acute Myocardial Infarction and Coronary Artery Disease) 2, edited by Jacob Haft, M.D. 265:283, 1978. Futura Publishing Co., Inc. Mt. Kisco, N.Y.

Kent, K.M. et al. "The Natural History of Asymptomatic or Mildly Symptomatic Patients with Coronary Artery Disease," Cardiology Branch, NHLBI, National Institutes of Health.

Lawrie, G.M. et al. "Results of Coronary Bypass at Least 10 Years after Operation in 250 Patients," *American Journal of Cardiology* 47:485, February 1981.

Loop, F.D. et al. "The Efficacy of Coronary Artery Surgery." *American Heart Journal* 101: 86–96, January 1981.

MacAlpin, R.N. et al. "Angina Pectoris at Rest with Preservation of Exercise Capacity. Prinzmetal's Variant Angina," *Circulation* 47:946–58, 1973.

Mathur, V.S. et al. "Prolonging Life with Coronary Bypass Surgery in Patients with Three-Vessel Disease," *Circulation* 62 (suppl. I) I–90–98, 1980.

McNeer, J.F. et al. "The Nature of Treatment Selection in Coronary Artery Disease," *Circulation* XLIX:606–14, April 1974.

Murphy, M.L. et al. "Treatment of Chronic Stable Angina," *New England Journal of Medicine* 297:620–26, Sept. 22, 1977.

Podrid, P.J. et al. "Prognosis of Medically Treated Patients with Coronary-Artery Disease with Profound ST-Segment Depression During Exercise Testing," *New England Journal of Medicine* 305:1111–16, Nov. 5, 1981.

Oberman, A. et al. "Natural History of Coronary Artery Disease," *Bulletin of New York Academy of Medicine* 48:1109–25, 1972.

Rosati, R.A. et al. "Does Coronary Surgery Prolong Life in Comparison with Medical Management?" *Postgraduate Medical Journal* 52:749–56, 1976.

Sandiford, F.M. et al. "The Aortocoronary Bypass Operation: Myth and Reality. An Overview Based on 10,000 Operations at the Texas Heart Institute," *International Surgery* 63:83–89, May–June 1978.

Sheldon, W.C. et al. "A Critique of the VA Cooperative Study," *Cleveland Clinic Quarterly* 45:225–30, 1978.

———. "Bypass Graft Surgery for Coronary Artery Disease: A 10–13 Year Follow-up Study of 741 Patients," *The American Journal of Cardiology* 47:485, February 1981.

Shubrooks, S.J. et al. "Variant Angina Pectoris. Clinical and Anatomic Spectrum and Result of Coronary Bypass Surgery," *American Journal of Cardiology* 36:142–47, 1975.

Silverman, M.E., and Flamm, M.D. "Variant Angina Pectoris. Anatomic Findings and Prognostic Implications," *Annals of Internal Medicine* 75:339–43, 1971.

"VA Cooperative Study Finds Bypass Improves Survival in New Cohort," *Journal of the American Medical Association* 243:1609, Apr. 25, 1980.

Wukasch, D.C. et al. "Surgical versus Medical Treatment of Coronary Artery Disease. Nine Year Follow-up of 9,061 Patients," *American Journal of Surgery* 137:201–07, 1978.

Zimmern, S.H. et al. "Total Occlusion of the Left Main Coronary Artery: The CASS Experience," *The American Journal of Cardiology* 47:408, February 1981.

☰ GLOSSARY

Afterload: The pressure against which the heart has to pump when it first starts to contract.

Aneurysm: The abnormal dilitation of a blood vessel, usually an artery, caused by a weakness in the vessel wall. In cardiac conditions, it refers to a scarred area of the heart that can hold a large amount of blood.

Angina Pectoris: The symptoms of coronary artery disease. Chest pain or discomfort, often extending to the arm, shoulder or jaw, which signifies that the heart muscle is not receiving enough blood.

Angiogram: An x-ray study of a blood vessel which follows the course of a radiopaque substance injected into the bloodstream. A cardiac angiogram reveals the extent and location of blockages in the coronary arteries.

Angiography: Also called angiocardiography. A method of visualizing the coronary arteries and pinpointing the locations and extent of blockages. Dye is injected into the coronary arteries through a catheter, and its path is traced to indicate location, extent and pattern of any blockages.

Angioplasty: The simple term sometimes used to describe Percutaneous Transluminal Coronary Angioplasty, the compression of blockages in the coronary arteries by passing a catheter through them.

Aorta: The main artery of the body which receives blood from the lower left chamber of the heart.

Arrhythmias: Irregular or abnormal heartbeats.

Arteriography: X rays of an artery which are taken after the injection of a radiopaque dye.

Arteriosclerosis: Thickening and loss of elasticity in the walls of arteries.

Atherosclerosis: The buildup of fatty and fibrous material in the inner linings of arteries that carry blood to the heart muscle. Arteries become clogged and blood supply is reduced.

Autonomic Nervous System: Regulator of involuntary functions such as breathing and heart action.

Beta-Blocker: A drug used to relieve angina pectoris.

Calcium Antagonist: A new category of drugs that blocks the uptake of calcium by the myocardial cells, dilates the coronary arteries and relieves the symptoms of angina pectoris.

Cardiac Catheterization: Examining the heart by introducing a catheter into a vein or artery and passing it through the heart.

Cardiac Index: The output of the heart corrected for body size.

Catecholamines: Substances called norepinephrine and epinephrine, produced by the adrenal glands. Norepinephrine increases the heartbeat rate and constricts muscle cells in the blood vessel walls. Epinephrine causes blood vessels in the skeletal muscles to relax which, in turn, increases the flow of blood to the muscles during exercise.

Chelation Therapy: A technique approved in the United States to treat heavy metal poisoning. Some practitioners say it can be used to treat coronary artery disease.

Cholesterol: A fatty substance which is produced by the body and which can be increased by intake of cholesterol-containing food. Many experts believe that there is a close relationship between cholesterol levels and coronary artery disease.

Chronic Stable Angina: Angina pain that has persisted for six months or more unchanged in intensity and controlled by medication.

Claudication: Pain in the leg vessels after walking certain distances, caused by defective circulation of the blood in the leg vessels.

Cold Potassium Cardioplegia: A solution that is injected into the aorta through a catheter during bypass surgery, and goes into the coronary arteries with the purpose of preserving the store of energy in the muscular wall of the heart during surgery.

Collateral Circulation: The way the body may compensate when large vessels are blocked. The body may build up channels—collaterals—through which blood can flow.

Costochondritis: Inflammation of the rib cage.

Distal Runoff: The area of the coronary artery beyond the obstruction.

Diuretics: Drugs which promote the excretion of urine, often used in the treatment of hypertension and congestive heart failure.

Echocardiogram: A method of diagnosing certain heart problems (for instance, valve disease). Ultrasound is transmitted into the body and the echoes returning from the surface of the heart are electronically plotted and recorded.

Ejection Fraction: A measurement of the pumping capacity of the heart muscle. It is a measure that can be obtained through a nuclear test (ventriculogram) or during catheterization.

Electrocardiogram: The written record of a test that amplifies the electrical charges in the contracting heart muscle. The test results, which look like squiggly lines on a long sheet of paper, reveal valuable information about heart rhythm and the electrical events within the heart muscle.

End Diastolic Pressure: Measurement of the pressure at the end of the diastolic phase of heart pumping when the heart is most relaxed. It is a reading taken during catheterization and helps determine the health of the heart muscle.

Esophagitis: Inflammation of the lining of the esophagus.

Familial Hypercholesterolemia: High levels of cholesterol in the blood that runs in families.

Hyperlipidemia: The term used to describe persons with high levels of fats in their blood.

Hypertension: High blood pressure.

Hypertrophic Cardiomyopathy: A condition in which the wall between the left and right ventricles of the heart becomes enlarged and obstructs the blood flow from the left ventricle. In more than half of patients with the condition, it is hereditary.

Hypoglycemia: Low blood sugar.

Hypothermia: A method of lowering body temperature during bypass surgery by cooling the blood going from the heart-lung machine to the patient.

Internal Mammary Artery: An artery which carries blood to the chest wall.

Intraaortic Balloon Pump: A device which helps a weakened heart pump fresh blood; a balloon inflates at the tip of a catheter which snakes up into the aorta from its point of insertion in a leg artery. It helps reduce the load on the heart, enabling it to work less.

Ischemia: A local deficiency of oxygen (usually brief), usually caused by an obstruction in or constriction of a blood vessel or vessels.

Labile Hypertension: Blood pressure that varies frequently.

Left Ventricular Aneurysm: A scarred area of the heart which can hold a lot of blood.

Left Ventricular Hypertrophy: Thickening of the left ventricle muscle because of an increased pressure load on the ventricle. A possible cause is high blood pressure.

Leukocytes: White blood cells.

Lipids: Fats and fatty substances.

Lipoproteins: a combination of fat (lipid) and protein molecules bound together.

Myocardial Infarction: Heart attack.

Myocardial Revascularization: Medical terminology for coronary bypass surgery.

Myocardium: Heart muscle.

Nitroglycerin: A medication used in the treatment of angina pectoris.

Nuclear Study: Diagnostic test effected through the injection of radioactive isotopes into the bloodstream and the charting of their course through specific areas of the body.

Nuclear Ventriculogram: A diagnostic procedure that reveals the wall motion of the heart's left ventricle and gives the patient's ejection fraction.

Partial Ileal Bypass: An operation on the intestines that reduces the amount of cholesterol that circulates through the blood.

Percutaneous Transluminal Coronary Angioplasty (PTCA): The compression of blockages in the coronary arteries by passing a catheter through them.

Pericarditis: A painful inflammation of the membrane surrounding the heart.

Peripheral Bruits: Turbulence in an artery usually caused by plaque in a vessel.

Prognostigram: A computer analysis of a patient's medical characteristics. It may help predict the course of his condition with or without surgery.

Prospective Randomized Study: A study in which patients, during a given time period, are assigned, at random, to a specific form of therapy (which may sometimes be no therapy at all) to reveal the outcome of each.

Prinzmetal's Variant Angina: A phenomenon whereby mysterious spasms temporarily constrict coronary arteries that are not clogged, and cause pain.

Retrospective Matched Study: A study which reviews previously observed patients.

Saphenous Veins: Veins in the leg which are used to accomplish coronary bypass surgery.

Septum: The wall of the heart.

Sphygmomanometer: The device used to measure blood pressure.

Spirometer: An instrument which measures the amount of air a person can hold in his or her lungs and the force with which it can be expelled.

Stable Angina: Anginal pain that has persisted for a long time —six months or more—unchanged in intensity and controlled by medication.

Stepped Care: The term used to describe stages of therapy.

Sternum: The breastbone.

Stress Test: A measurement of the heart's ability to deliver blood containing oxygen to the heart muscles as they work harder and harder. The patient's heart, pulse rate and blood pressure are monitored as he exercises on a bicycle or treadmill.

Triglyceride: A fat in the blood that may have a relationship to coronary artery disease.

Unstable Angina: Intense and prolonged angina while resting with little or no response to medication; angina that has increased in frequency and intensity in the past three months; angina experienced within 30 days after a heart attack, and new angina.

Variant Angina: See Prinzmetal's angina.

Vasodilator: Drug which relaxes the muscles of the arteries. It is used in treating high blood pressure and other ailments.

Ventricular Gallop: Heart sound that is often the first sign of congestive heart failure.

INDEXES

Subject Index

339

Name Index